POCKET CONSL

Infection

R.T.D. Emond
MB, ChB, FRCP, DTM&H
Consulting Physician
The Royal Free Hospital
London

J.M. Bradley
MB, BS, FRCPath
Consulting Microbiologist
The Royal Free Hospital
London

N.S. Galbraith
CBE, MB, BS, FRCP, FFCM
Formerly Director
Communicable Diseases Surveillance Centre
Public Health Laboratory Service
London

SECOND EDITION

OXFORD

Blackwell Scientific Publications

LONDON EDINBURGH BOSTON

MELBOURNE PARIS BERLIN VIENNA

©1982, 1989 by
Blackwell Scientific Publications
Editorial offices:
Osney Mead, Oxford OX2 0EL
25 John Street, London WC1N 2BL
23 Ainslie Place, Edinburgh EH3 6AJ
3 Cambridge Center, Cambridge,
    Massachusetts 02142, USA
54 University Street, Carlton
    Victoria 3053, Australia

Other Editorial Offices:
Arnette SA
2, rue Casimir-Delavigne
75006 Paris
France

Blackwell Wissenschaft
Meinekestrasse 4
D-1000 Berlin 15
Germany

Blackwell MZV
Feldgasse 13
A-1238 Wien
Austria

First published 1982
Reprinted 1984
Spanish edition 1984
Second edition 1989
Reprinted 1991

Set by Setrite Typesetters, Hong Kong
Printed and bound in Great Britain
by Billings and Sons Ltd, Worcester

DISTRIBUTORS

Marston Book Services Ltd
PO Box 87
Oxford OX2 0DT
(*Orders*: Tel: 0865 791155
         Fax: 0865 791927
         Telex: 837515)

USA
Mosby-Year Book, Inc.
11830 Westline Industrial Drive
St Louis, Missouri 63146
(*Orders*: Tel: 800 633-6699)

Canada
Mosby-Year Book, Inc.
5240 Finch Avenue East
Scarborough, Ontario
(*Orders*: Tel: 416 298 1588)

Australia
Blackwell Scientific Publications
(Australia) Pty Ltd
54 University Street
Carlton, Victoria 3053
(*Orders*: Tel: 03 347 0300)

British Library
Cataloguing in Publication Data

Edmond, R.T.D.
    Infection. — 2nd ed.
1. Man. Communicable diseases
I. Title II. Bradley, J.M.
III. Galbraith, N.S.
616.9

ISBN 0-632-02163-2

Contents

Preface to second edition, vii

Actinomycosis, 1
Anaerobic infections, 3
    Non-sporing anaerobes, 3
    Sporing anaerobes, 4
Anthrax, 8
Arthritis, 11
    Aseptic (non-suppurative), 11
    Septic (suppurative), 12
Aspergillosis, 15

Brucellosis, 18

Candida infections, 21
Cat-scratch fever, 24
Chancroid, 26
Chlamydial infections, 28
    Chlamydia trachomatis, 28
    Chlamydia psittaci, 32
Cholera, 35
Colitis, 38
    Haemorrhagic, 38
    Necrotizing enterocolitis in infants, 39
    Pseudomembranous, 40
Congenital and neonatal infections, 43
Conjunctivitis, 47
    Specific syndromes, 47
    Non-specific syndromes, 49
Cytomegalovirus infection, 52

Dengue, 55
Diphtheria, 57
Dysentery, 61
    Amoebic, 61
    Bacillary, 64
    Schistosomal, 66

Contents

Encephalitis, 69
Endocarditis (infective), 73
Enterovirus infections, 77

Food poisoning, 83
    Botulism, 83
    Staphylococcal, 85
    Bacillus cereus, 86
    Clostridium perfringens, 87
    Salmonella (*see* salmonella infections, p. 246)
    Vibrio parahaemolyticus, 89
    Viral, 90
    Toxic substances, 91

Gastroenteritis, 94
    Campylobacter, 94
    Escherichia coli, 96
    Viral, 99
    Cryptosporidial, 101
Giardiasis, 104
Gonorrhoea, 106

Haemolytic uraemic syndrome, 110
Haemophilus influenzae infections, 112
Helminth infections: common intestinal helminths, 115
Hepatitis (viral), 120
Herpes simplex infections, 129
HIV infection, 133

Infectious mononucleosis, 140
Influenza, 143

Kawasaki disease (mucocutaneous lymph node syndrome), 147

Legionella infection, 149
    Legionnaires disease, 149
    Pontiac fever, 152
Leptospirosis, 153

Contents

Listeriosis, 157
Lyme disease, 160

Malaria, 163
Measles, 170
Meningitis, 174
    Aseptic, 174
    Septic, 178
Meningococcal infection, 182
Mumps, 186
Mycobacterial infections, 189
    Tuberculosis, 189
    Atypical mycobacteria, 196
    Leprosy, 198

Osteomyelitis, 202

Parvovirus B19 infections, 205
Pelvic inflammatory disease, 207
Pertussis, 209
Pneumonia, 212
    Acute bacterial, 212
    Primary atypical, 215
    Viral, 217
    Protozoal, 219
Post-abortum and post-partum sepsis, 222
Pyrexia of undetermined origin (PUO), 225

Q fever, 229

Rabies, 232
Respiratory infection (acute), 237
Rubella, 241

Salmonella infections, 246
    Infections other than typhoid or paratyphoid fevers, 246
    Typhoid and paratyphoid fevers (enteric fever), 250
Skin infections, 257

Contents

Bacterial, 257
Fungal, 262
Viral, 265
Parasitic, 268
Staphylococcal infections, 271
Streptococcal infections, 277
    Group A streptococci (*Strep. pyogenes*), 277
    Group B streptococci, 285
    Other species of streptococci, 287

Tetanus, 290
Toxoplasmosis, 295
Treponemal infections, 299
    Syphilis, 299
    Yaws, 304
Tularaemia, 307
Typhus, 309

Urinary tract infections, 315

Varicella (chickenpox) and herpes zoster (shingles), 321
Viral haemorrhagic fevers (VHF), 325
    Arthropod-borne, 325
    Zoonotic, 329
    Marburg and Ebola virus diseases, 331

Yersinia infections, 336
    Plague, 336
    Other infections, 339

Appendix A: Chemoprophylaxis, 342
Appendix B: Infection control, 346
Appendix C: Immunization, 352

Index, 367

Preface to second edition

The pattern of infection in most communities has changed radically with improvements in social and economic standards. Many endemic diseases of Europe and North America have been reduced to insignificant proportions. Nevertheless, infection still forms an important part of medical practice and many new problems have emerged as a result of the enormous expansion in air travel and the development of high-technology medicine, with its unwelcome legacy of the immune-impaired host.

We have endeavoured to summarize current knowledge of some of the common and more important infections in the community. In doing so we have placed particular emphasis on viral and bacterial infections, and have included a major section on the problems related to Aids. In this second edition we have expanded the sections on protozoal infections to include those conditions of importance to the traveller and have incorporated some of the intestinal helminth infections. In order to keep this volume to a pocket size we have of necessity been brief and may have left out topics relevant to some parts of the world. For this we seek the understanding and forbearance of the reader.

The book is arranged alphabetically and, except in a few instances when it has seemed logical to organize the information differently, each entry is divided into the following sections: organism, epidemiology, pathogenesis, clinical features, laboratory diagnosis, treatment and prevention. In some sections the material has been tabulated, in most it has not. We have adopted this structured system to assist the reader, who requires a *vade mecum* and will wish to consult this book frequently and readily.

R.T.D.E.
J.M.B.
N.S.G.

Actinomycosis

Organism
Actinomyces israeli: obligate parasite; anaerobic, Gram-positive rod.

Epidemiology

Distribution
Worldwide, sporadic, uncommon. About 150 inpatients per year
in UK and 1−2 deaths. Commonest in young adults; more frequent in males than females, and in agricultural workers than other
occupations.

Source
Human: part of normal flora around teeth, in tonsillar crypts and in
gastrointestinal tract.

Spread
Endogenous infection; often follows trauma. Cervicofacial disease
commonest form; may follow dental extraction. Abdominal disease
may follow surgical operations, such as appendicectomy. Pelvic
infection in females associated with IUDC; often symptomless.

Pathogenesis
Precise initiating factors not known. Organism stimulates granulomatous inflammatory response. Lesion extends by contiguity until
it reaches the surface where it presents as a firm mass, parts of which
break down to form sinuses; pus may contain sulphur granules
(aggregates of organism). Rarely dissemination by bloodstream.

Clinical features

Cervicofacial
Tender swelling about angle of jaw or ramus, affecting soft tissue
more than bone; progresses to abscesses and multiple sinuses.

Skin
Lesion primary or secondary to infection in deeper tissues; round,
firm swelling followed by ulceration.

Actinomycosis

Clinical features

Pulmonary
Cough, fever, haemoptysis; basal signs, pleural effusions; progressive lung infiltration; periostitis of ribs strongly suggestive.

Abdominal
Presents as acute appendicitis or slowly growing mass in right iliac fossa; spreads to adjacent structures.

CNS
Infection of brain by direct spread or as a result of pyaemia.

Laboratory diagnosis
- Initial diagnosis is clinical.
- Confirmation by microscopy and anaerobic culture of expressed pus or of dressing in contact with sinus for some hours; superficial swabs inadequate.
- Serological tests unhelpful.

Treatment
- Prolonged treatment with penicillin in high dosage with or without additional sulphonamides.
- Aminoglycoside or tetracycline as possible alternatives.
- Surgical treatment consists of drainage or incision and curettage.

Prevention

Immediate
- Isolation unnecessary.
- Contacts: no action.

Longterm
- Oral hygiene, especially following dental treatment.

Anaerobic infections

1 Non-sporing anaerobes

Organisms
Bacteroides and *Fusobacterium*: non-sporing, Gram-negative rods; obligate anaerobes. Species differentiation by biochemical tests, gas−liquid chromography (GLC) and antibiotic sensitivities. *B. fragilis*, *B. melaninogenicus* most frequent clinical isolates. In these circumstances, *B. fragilis* is capsulated and produces several exo-toxins, proteases, lipases and heparinases.

Anaerobic cocci (*Peptostreptococcus*, *Peptococcus*), strict anaerobes, rarely speciated in clinical laboratories. (CO_2-dependent streptococci found in similar situations, but these are facultative anaerobes).

Epidemiology

Distribution
Infections worldwide, sporadic, usually in debilitated persons. Bac-teroides and anaerobic streptococcal infections may act synergistically in giving rise to disease.

Source
Human: normal flora of oropharynx, gastrointestinal tract and female lower genital tract.

Spread
Endogenous infection usually follows tissue damage by accidental trauma or surgical operation, or by infection with aerobic bacteria and viruses, or occurs in tissues where oxygen tension is low be-cause of vascular disease. Not transmissible from patient to patient; very rarely from person to person by bites, contamination of fingers in health-care workers and by sharing of injection equipment in drug abusers.

Pathogenesis
Commonly several species of anaerobes, with or without aerobes, isolated from a single lesion; complex synergistic relationship highly probable.

Capsulation of *B. fragilis* enhances virulence and exotoxins probably important. Evidence to show that the anaerobic environment and some obligate anaerobes impair phagocytosis. Septic thrombotic phenomena, including metastatic infection, not uncommon.

Clinical features

Bacteroides and fusobacterium
Damage to gut wall or to genital tract, especially in immunodeficient patient. Foul-smelling purulent discharge from abscesses in any situation. Bacteraemia associated with severe chills and high remittent fever, often accompanied by shock. Uterine infection complicated by septic thrombophlebitis with secondary abscesses in liver or lung. Liver abscess, endocarditis and meningitis. Dental infection may spread to nasal sinuses, middle ear or brain.

Anaerobic cocci
Wound infection. Synergistic bacterial gangrene. Myositis. Cerebral abscess.

Laboratory diagnosis
See sporing anaerobes.

Treatment
See sporing anaerobes.

Prevention
See sporing anaerobes.

2 Sporing anaerobes

Organisms
Clostridium spp.: sporing, Gram-positive rods. Species differentiated biochemically and by GLC. Genus includes non-pathogenic species. Pathogenic species produce a variety of exotoxins. Species responsible for infections of tissues include: *Cl. perfringens (welchii), Cl. novyi (oedematiens), Cl. septicum, Cl. histolyticum, Cl. sordelli.* See also food poisoning: *Cl. perfringens*, p. 87 and *Cl. botulinum*, p. 83;

tetanus: *Cl. tetani*, p. 290; pseudomembranous colitis: *Cl. difficle*, p. 40.

Epidemiology

Distribution
Infections worldwide, usually sporadic. Gas gangrene formerly common in wounded soldiers, now rare in both military and civilian practice; may follow severe compound fractures or illegal abortion. Wound botulism very rare; may follow severe compound fractures or crush injuries to limbs; has been reported in intravenous drug abusers with infected lesions at injection sites.

Source
Organisms widely distributed in gastrointestinal tract of man and animals, in dust and soil.

Spread
Endogenous or contamination from environment of wounds where oxygen tension is low because of trauma, infection or defective blood supply. Not transmissible from person to person.

Pathogenesis
Multiplication of clostridia in favourable site accompanied by production of exotoxins; the alpha-toxin, a lecithinase, of *Cl. perfringens* has potential to damage cell membranes and intracellular structures. Other toxins include: lethal substances, deoxyribonuclease, hyaluronidase, proteinase. Metabolism of tissue carbohydrates produces gas and lowers pH, thus potentiating the anaerobic conditions.

Clinical features

Asymptomatic
Clostridia are found as surface contaminants in 30% of war wounds.

Mild local infection
Clostridia of low virulence invade the fascial planes producing gas in the tissues. Illness of gradual onset and benign course. No discolor-

ation of skin. X-ray may demonstrate impalpable gas in clostridial cellulitis or myositis.

Severe local infection
Infection with highly virulent strains produces extensive cellulitis with involvement of muscle and terminal (agonal) invasion of bloodstream. Increasing pain and surrounding oedema. Little fever but sharp rise in pulse rate and falling blood pressure. Serosanguineous discharge. Skin turns pale and black bullae form containing bloody fluid; bubbles of gas detected clinically or on radiography. Renal failure. General intoxication profound.

Bacteraemia
Intravascular haemolysis, anaemia, haemoglobinuria, anuria and jaundice.

Laboratory diagnosis
The diagnosis of these anaerobic infections is clinical; isolation of clostridia does not necessarily indicate infection, neither does isolation of *Bacteroides* spp. from sites with a commensal flora which includes anaerobes.
- Collection of adequate specimens is of paramount importance (aspirated pus, transported in 'gassed-out' tubes, is greatly preferable to swabs).
- Blood cultures should also be taken, including anaerobic medium such as thiol or thioglycollate.
- Good methodology, including selective media and anaerobiosis, important if infections are to be diagnosed adequately.
- Gas–liquid chromatography of pus, of inoculated cooked-meat medium, and of anaerobic blood culture often helpful in making early diagnosis of anaerobic infection by demonstration of typical patterns of volatile fatty acids.

Treatment
The best results are obtained by surgical drainage combined with antibacterial therapy using, in the UK, metronidazole, or in the USA, clindamycin, along with gentamicin or another appropriate drug for concomitant aerobic infection.

Prevention

Immediate
- Isolation usually unnecessary but see pseudomembranous colitis, p. 42.
- Inform hospital control-of-infection officer.
- Epidemiological and environmental investigation if there is a possibility of an environmental source of sporing anaerobes.

Longterm
- Treatment of primary condition.
- Careful preoperative preparation in elective gastrointestinal, pelvic and lower limb surgery, including prophylactic chemotherapy.
- Wound surgery to remove damaged and devitalized tissue; prophylactic chemotherapy.

Anthrax

Organism

Bacillus anthracis: large Gram-positive aerobic, spore-bearing rod; the only virulent pathogen in a genus of which other species are ubiquitous and free-living. The anthrax bacillus is capsulated and produces a protein exotoxin complex.

Epidemiology

Distribution

Worldwide zoonosis, endemic in areas where animal infection is common, rare sporadic infection in industrialized countries. Less than ten cases of cutaneous anthrax reported in UK 1980−87.

Source

Usually cattle, sheep or goats. Spores remain viable for many years in animal products (hair, hides and bone meal) and in environment (dust, pastureland).

Spread

Non-industrial anthrax (cutaneous): direct contact in farmers, butchers, veterinarians and others handling infected animals or contaminated animal products. Industrial anthrax (pulmonary and cutaneous): inhalation and direct contact in workers processing hair, wool, hides and bone. Ingestion giving rise to gastrointestinal anthrax rare. Person-to-person transmission has not been reported.

Pathogenesis

The virulent organism proliferates at the site of entry: bacteria are numerous beneath the central necrotic area of skin lesion. Capsule and exotoxin inhibit phagocytosis. Bacteraemia may follow primary infection at any site.

Clinical features

Incubation is generally 48 hours but may extend from 1−10 days.

Cutaneous anthrax (malignant pustule, hide porters' disease)
- *Local lesion*: painless area of necrosis surrounded by haemor-

rhagic vesicles and indurated zone of oedema, progressing to thick
dark leathery scab followed by deep ulceration. Occasionally inflammatory oedema without focal lesion.
- *General*: fever, headache and joint pains. Occasionally septicaemia
and meningitis: polymorphonuclear leucocytosis.

Pulmonary anthrax
Fulminating attack of pneumonia with frequent haemoptyses.

Intestinal anthrax
Acute gastroenteritis with bloody diarrhoea, very rare in man.

Laboratory diagnosis
The organism can be demonstrated microscopically in material
obtained from the undersurface of the eschar, but culture and
identification by appropriate biochemical tests must be performed to
differentiate it from the many non-pathogenic *Bacillus* spp.

Treatment
Benzylpenicillin 300 mg i.m. 6-hourly for 5−7 days.

Prevention

Immediate
- Isolation: cutaneous anthrax — wound precautions; pulmonary —
respiratory precautions in infectious diseases unit. Incineration of
contaminated material.
- Early specific chemotherapy.
- Identify contacts exposed to same source.
- Surveillance of contacts for 7 days after exposure. Early specific
treatment if symptoms develop. Prophylactic chemotherapy may be
considered for persons heavily exposed, such as veterinarians who
have carried out an autopsy on an animal later suspected of dying
from anthrax. (Benzylpenicillin 600 mg i.m. in one dose and
benzathine penicillin 916 mg i.m. in one dose.)
- Report to health authority; notifiable in UK.
- Investigate source and spread.
- Report animal infection to agricultural authority.

Longterm
- Immunization of animals in endemic areas.
- Disposal of infected carcasses by incineration or burial in lime.
- Disinfection or sterilization of animal products.
- Protection of workers in hazardous industries: dust control, ventilation of industrial premises, protective clothing, waterproof dressings for skin injuries.
- Immunization of workers at risk (p. 362).

Arthritis

1 Aseptic (non-suppurative)

Organism/disease	Epidemiology	Pathogenesis
Numerous systemic infections including: Meningococcal disease	Immediately follows acute phase, or forms component of chronic bacteraemia	Immune-complex deposition in acute meningococcal infection. Possibly other aseptic arthritides have similar aetiology
Salmonella infection	See p. 246	Associated with HLA-B27 in salmonella, shigella and yersinia infections
Shigella infection	See p. 64	
Yersinia infection	See p. 339	
Brucellosis	See p. 18	
Syphilis	See p. 299	
Lyme disease	See p. 160	
Rubella	Commonest in females after puberty; rarely affects males	Endocrine factor in women for rubella and in men for mumps.
Mumps	More common in males than in females	
Virus B hepatitis	See p. 121	
Parvovirus B19 infection	Common complication, particularly in adults	

Clinical features

Meningococcal arthritis
- One or two large joints involved in acute infection.

Clinical features

- Polyarthritis in chronic disease.
- Septic arthritis may occur.

Salmonella, shigella and yersinia infections
- Usually develops within 2 weeks of onset of diarrhoea.
- Involves large joints of lower limbs and small joints of upper limbs.

Virus infections
- Usually polyarthritis.
- Associated tenosynovitis in rubella.
- Parvovirus arthritis usually transient but may persist for several months.

Laboratory diagnosis
- Look for evidence of primary disease.
- Essential to exclude septic arthritis (p. 14)
- *Joint aspirate*:
  Cytology: $<50\,000$ WBC/mm^3; polymorphonuclear cells may predominate.
  Culture: must be performed but expected to be sterile.

Treatment
- Aspirin or non-steroidal anti-inflammatory drug.
- Rarely corticosteroid intra-articularly.

2 Septic (suppurative)

Organism	Epidemiology	Pathogenesis
Staph. aureus	Commonest cause in children over 2 years	Predisposing causes: trauma, corticosteroid therapy, diabetes mellitus, rheumatoid and osteoarthritis, immunodeficiency, endocrine function (e.g. menstruation and
Streptococci, including *S. pneumoniae*	See p. 277	
Neisseria gonorrhoeae	See p. 106	

Arthritis: Septic (suppurative)

Organism/epidemiology/pathogenesis

Organism	Epidemiology	Pathogenesis
Haemophilus influenzae	Predominant cause in children under 2 years	pregnancy in gonococcal arthritis)
Enterobacteria, including salmonellae, especially *Salm. cholerae-suis*	Salmonella infection derived from animals, *Salm. cholerae-suis* from pigs	Entry of organism via: • direct wound • spread from contiguous tissues • bloodstream
Pseudomonas aeruginosa	Particularly common in drug addicts	
Mycobacterium tuberculosis and *M. bovis*	Commonly caused by *M. bovis* derived from infected cattle by consumption of contaminated milk and dairy products. In countries with tuberculosis-free herds and pasteurization of milk the disease is rare and nearly always caused by *M. tuberculosis*	See p. 190

Clinical features

General features
- Usually a single joint affected, commonly the knee.
- Acute onset except in tuberculous infection.
- Painful, hot, swollen joint with effusion in acute infections.
- Constitutional disturbance.

Specific features
Gonorrhoea and tuberculosis are important causes of arthritis, involving small joints of hands and wrists.
- *Gonococcal arthritis*: usually a polyarthritis, petechial or vesicular

Clinical features

rash common, tenosynovitis in some cases. May be very similar to meningococcal arthritis (p. 183).

● *Tuberculous arthritis*: more chronic presentation, commonly involves weight-bearing joints, may be associated with tenosynovitis (p. 203)

Laboratory diagnosis
● Blood cultures should always be taken.
● Search for primary source of infection.
● *Joint aspirate*:
Cytology: >50 000 WBC/mm^3: >90% polymorphonuclear cells in acute infection.
Culture: on appropriate media for recovery of all likely pathogens, including mycobacteria if clinical features suggestive; antibiotic sensitivities must be determined.

Treatment
● Avoid weight bearing until infection subsides.
● Repeated aspiration or surgical drainage may be required occasionally.
● *Neonates*: penicillinase-resistant penicillin plus gentamicin.
Children under 2 years: ampicillin, amoxycillin, chloramphenicol or co-trimoxazole.
● *Older children and adults*: penicillinase-resistant penicillin, clindamycin or sodium fusidate.
● *Gonococcal arthritis*: benzylpenicillin for 3−5 days or tetracycline.
● *Pseudomonas arthritis*: gentamicin, carbenicillin or cephalosporin according to sensitivity of organism.
● *Tuberculous arthritis*: ethambutol and isoniazid with or without rifampicin.
● *Duration of treatment*: acute, 6 weeks; chronic, 12 weeks; tuberculous, 12 months.

Aspergillosis

Organism
Aspergilli are ubiquitous filamentous fungi, readily cultured on appropriate media, and characterized morphologically. *A. fumigatus* is an opportunistic pathogen; other species rarely cause disease.

Epidemiology

Distribution
Infection worldwide, sporadic, uncommon. Most often seen in immuno-compromised or other susceptible persons.

Source
Widely distributed in environment. Grows on decaying vegetable matter.

Spread
Airborne, inhalation of spores. Not transmissible from person to person.

Pathogenesis
• Aspergilloma (fungus ball) occurs in previously damaged lung, e.g. in bronchiectasis; there is no invasion of surrounding tissues but blood vessel erosion may cause repeated haemoptyses.
• Necrotizing bronchopneumonia occurs in the immunocompromised; at autopsy vascular invasion and wide dissemination of fungus may be demonstrable.
• Allergic pulmonary aspergillosis may occur without evidence of preceding lung disease.

Clinical features

Lungs
• Aspergilloma usually discovered accidentally on X-ray examination. Solitary lesion in upper lobe. Usually symptomless but may cause fever and haemoptysis.
• Allergic bronchopulmonary infiltration gives rise to recurrent attacks of fever, chest discomfort and wheezing.

Aspergillosis

Clinical features

- Acute and usually fatal pneumonia in immunosuppressed. Haematogenous spread.

Central nervous system (CNS)
Cerebral infarction in immunosuppressed; brain abscess in normal patient.

Heart
Endocarditis in normal heart or after valve replacement.

Eye
Keratitis; endophthalmitis in immunosuppressed.

Ear, nose and throat (ENT)
- Benign infection of external auditory canal, especially after prolonged use of antibacterial eardrops.
- Fungus ball in sinus.
- Invasive sinusitis.

Laboratory diagnosis

Culture
Aspergilli are common saprophytic fungi, therefore diagnosis should not be based solely on positive culture. Fungal elements should also be seen in biopsy specimens, bronchial aspirate, or in sputum.

Serology
Specific antibodies, demonstrable by agar precipitation, complement fixation, immunoelectrophoresis or indirect fluorescent antibody techniques, detectable in aspergilloma and allergic pulmonary infection; diagnosis by serology or culture not always successful.

Treatment

Medical
- Amphotericin B 0.25−1.5 mg/kg daily i.v. possibly in combination with flucytosine or rifampicin, may be used for severe or disseminated infection.

Aspergillosis

Treatment

- Otitis externa: nystatin by insufflation, or clioquinol or neomycin undecenoate applied on gauze wick.

Surgical
Excision of circumscribed lesion and removal of infected prosthesis.

Prevention

Immediate
- Isolation unnecessary.
- Contacts: no action.
- Report to hospital control-of-infection officer.
- Investigation of source of nosocomial infections.

Longterm
- In hospitals: air filtration to prevent spores entering environment of highly susceptible patients.

Brucellosis

Organisms
Brucellae: aerobic, Gram-negative coccobacilli which primarily infect a wide range of animals. Two species, *B. abortus* and *B. melitensis*, are the principal human pathogens; infections with *B. suis* occur occasionally, and with *B. canis* rarely.

Epidemiology

Distribution
Zoonosis. Endemic in Mediterranean, Asia, Central and South America; rare in North America, North West Europe; in UK 20–30 cases per year 1980–87, over half imported. Sporadic occupational cases (farmers, veterinarians, abattoir workers), occasional outbreaks due to milk or dairy products.

Source
Cattle (*B. abortus*): UK, North West Europe. Sheep and goats (*B. melitensis*): Mediterranean. Rarely pigs (*B. suis*) and dogs (*B. canis*).

Spread
Direct contact with products of conception of infected animals. Inhalation, working in confined spaces with animals at parturition. Consumption of unpasteurized milk or dairy products. Accidental self-inoculation of live vaccines in veterinarians. Person-to-person spread virtually unknown.

Pathogenesis
The organisms are ingested by and multiply within polymorphonuclear leucocytes which subsequently lyse, liberating the bacteria. If the infection is not overcome at this stage the brucellae disseminate and localize within cells in organs such as the spleen, liver or bones where they stimulate a granulomatous response.

The intermittent liberation of viable organisms, or their breakdown products, is thought to be responsible for the periodicity of symptoms.

In addition to the cell-mediated immune response, humoral antibodies are formed.

Clinical features

Incubation
Usually 2−4 weeks, but may be several months.

Acute brucellosis
- Onset: sudden or gradual.
- *Pattern of illness*: not sharply defined; extremes ambulant or fulminating; commonest pattern undulant with febrile periods followed by apyrexial periods, rise of temperature in afternoon.
- *Major features*: fatigue, drenching sweats, pains in limbs and arthralgia or arthritis; nervousness, insomnia and depression; enlargement of liver and spleen; multisystem involvement in fulminating cases.

Chronic brucellosis
- May develop insidiously or follow acute attack.
- Often a history of recurrent bouts of fever accompanied by sweating, lassitude, headache, pain in back and limbs.
- Few physical signs though splenomegaly may be present in 10% of cases.
- Condition may remain undiagnosed for years and symptoms attributed to neurosis.

Hypersensitivity
Veterinarians may become hypersensitive to brucella antigen and develop a skin rash or febrile illness as a result of exposure to infected animals. This does not necessarily imply chronic brucellosis.

Laboratory diagnosis

Acute infection
- Blood cultures, in Liquoid broth or a diphasic medium, incubated in air plus 5−10% CO_2, may be positive during the acute phase of infections; they should be incubated for at least 6 weeks.
- Total white cell count is normally less than 7×10^9/litre; a polymorphonuclear leucocytosis makes the diagnosis virtually untenable.
- Serology: IgM antibodies are detectable from the second week

of the illness. Antigens prepared from both *B. abortus* and *B. melitensis* should be used even in suspected *B. abortus* infections as some biotypes of the latter have predominant melitensis-type antigenic structure.

Subacute and chronic infection
- Blood cultures are seldom positive.
- IgM antibodies may not be found.
- IgG antibodies are usually detected but may occasionally be absent in confirmed cases. Tests for IgG antibody include antihuman globulin (Coomb's), complement fixation and radioimmunoassay.
- Brucellin skin test, demonstrating cell-mediated hypersensitivity, is rarely of diagnostic significance.
- Serological testing in all forms of brucellosis must be interpreted in conjunction with the clinical picture and should be performed in experienced laboratories.

Treatment
- Tetracycline orally in a dosage of 0.5 g 6-hourly for a min. of 6 weeks.
- When attack is severe this may be combined with streptomycin 1 g daily by i.m. injection for the first 3 weeks.
- Acute attacks respond satisfactorily but chronic brucellosis responds poorly. Further courses may be required.

Prevention

Immediate
- Isolation unnecessary.
- Investigate source and spread.
- Contacts: identify persons exposed to same source so that those infected may be treated.
- Report to health authority.
- Report animal infection to agricultural authority.

Longterm
- Eradication of infection in farm animals.
- Vaccination of animals.
- Pasteurization of milk and dairy products.

Candida infections

Organism

Candida spp.: yeast-like fungi. The species most commonly infecting man is *Candida albicans*, a minor component of the commensal flora in the mouth, gastrointestinal tract, vagina and sometimes skin.

Epidemiology

Distribution

Infection worldwide. Oral thrush common in infants. Frequent cause of vulvovaginitis in women. Common in patients with Aids; other predisposing factors include pregnancy, diabetes, debility, immuno-suppression, chemotherapy and use of oral contraceptives.

Source
Human: cases or carriers.

Spread
Endogenous infection common. Direct contact with infected person. Environmental contamination, especially in nurseries.

Pathogenesis

Majority of candida infections involve superficial tissues where there is some disturbance of local defences. Systemic invasion is rare and found only in severely ill or immunocompromised individuals, especially after broad-spectrum antibiotic therapy.

Clinical features

Oral
- *Acute pseudomembranous (thrush)*: white papules or cotton-wool patches on erythematous base.
- *Acute atrophic*: painful mouth, smooth erythematous tongue, angular stomatitis.
- *Chronic hypertrophic*: firm diffuse white plaques or numerous white papules with intervening erythema. May persist for many years.
- *Chronic atrophic (denture stomatitis)*: diffuse erythema on palate under dentures. Usually symptomless.

Clinical features

Cutaneous
- *Intertrigo*: common condition affecting moist skin folds. Skin erythematous and macerated.
- *Paronychia*: infection may spread from the nail fold under the adjacent nail causing deformity and even loss of the nail.
- *Nappy rash*: starts around anus and spreads over perineum affecting areas in contact with nappy. Skin reddened and macerated.

Mucocutaneous
- *Chronic localized*: starts in childhood with oral candidiasis which persists and spreads to nails and skin of hands and feet.
- *Chronic localized with granulomata*: similar to above but with granulomatous lesions on face and scalp. Starts in infancy.
- *Chronic localized with endocrine disorder*: children and young adults, familial tendency, usually preceding endocrine disturbance or pernicious anaemia.

Genital
- *Vaginitis*: pruritus, scanty or thick white discharge, redness of vagina and labia.
- *Balanitis*: severe irritation, blisters and patches of thrush.

Deep tissues
- *Central nervous system*: encephalitis, meningitis.
- *Heart*: endocarditis, myocarditis, pericarditis.
- *Lungs*: pneumonia, no characteristic features.
- *Urinary tract*: symptomless cystitis or pyelonephritis.
- *Eye*: postoperative or haematogenous spread, any structure affected.

Systemic or disseminated (candidosis)
- *Immunocompromised patients*: multi-organ involvement, especially of heart, kidney, brain and eye. Multiple small abscesses: blood cultures not always positive. Difficult to diagnose.

Laboratory diagnosis
- Gram-stained clinical material for yeast cells and pseudohyphae.
- Culture on Sabouraud's agar or other simple media.

Laboratory diagnosis

- Blood cultures are preferably taken into a special medium (Sabouraud broth or Myocult). Organisms isolated from the blood should be fully identified by fermentation and assimilation tests.
- Detection of antigenaemia, e.g. by latex fixation, useful in deep tissue and disseminated infections.

Treatment

Systemic
- Flucytosine alone or in combination with amphotericin. Resistance to flucytosine not uncommon, so sensitivity testing essential before treatment. Regular liver function tests and blood counts.
- Amphotericin not absorbed from gut and must be given parenterally. Toxic to kidney, so renal function tests essential. Synergistic with flucytosine.
- Imidazole-based compounds, such as ketoconazole and miconazole, are toxic and have been associated with liver damage and hypersensitivity reactions so require careful monitoring. Not first choice.

Prevention

Immediate
- Isolation: wound precautions in nurseries.
- Treatment of underlying condition.
- Early detection and treatment of cases in nurseries and hospitals.
- Inform hospital control-of-infection officer.

Longterm
- Care of mucous membranes in susceptible subjects.
- Early detection and treatment of infection.

Cat-scratch fever

Organism
Pleomorphic short rods demonstrated by silver-impregnation methods applied to skin and lymph node biopsies; stain as Gram-negative with modified Gram stain; found free and within macrophages; not yet cultured.

Epidemiology
Rare disease. Mainly affects children and young adults. Associated with scratch, bite or lick of cat or other animal; cats show no evidence of disease.

Pathogenesis
Necrotic foci appear in germinal follicles of lymph nodes and break down to form microabscesses. Foci surrounded by layer of epithelioid cells interspersed by giant cells of Langhans type. Vigorous cell-mediated hypersensitivity reaction occurs after intradermal injection of material prepared from infected tissue.

Clinical features
- Primary lesion appears at site of injury.
- Progressive enlargement of regional lymph nodes after 10−30 days.
- Headache, malaise and low-grade fever: occasional rashes.
- Suppuration and discharging sinus in severe attacks.
- Resolves over period of 2−12 weeks.
- Rarely encephalitis, myelitis or radiculitis.
- Specific skin test; skin sensitivity may persist for many years.

Laboratory diagnosis
This is directed towards exclusion of other infections, especially tularaemia, toxoplasmosis and infectious mononucleosis (see p. 307, 297 and 142).

Treatment
Antibiotics are ineffective. Repeated aspiration or surgical drainage of abscess.

Prevention

Immediate
- Isolation unnecessary.
- Thorough cleansing of animal bites and scratches.

Longterm
- None.

Chancroid

Organism
Haemophilus ducreyi; small Gram-negative rod; *in vitro* culture difficult.

Epidemiology

Distribution
Infection worldwide, common in tropics and subtropics, rare in temperate zones. About 80 reported cases per year in UK 1980−86. May be associated with heterosexual spread of HIV, especially in sub-Saharan Africa.

Source
Human: lesions of genital tract, which may be symptomless in women; discharging lesions on the skin.

Spread
Sexual contact. Direct contact with pus from lesion.

Pathogenesis
H. ducreyi cannot penetrate intact skin but invades via small abrasions and multiplies in the dermis, inciting an inflammatory response. The resulting pustule ruptures, forming a shallow ulcer. Inflammation also in regional lymph nodes but uncommon to demonstrate *H. ducreyi* in nodes. A cell-mediated immune response is detectable, but does not protect against reinfection.

Clinical features
- Incubation period: 1−21 days.
- Initial lesions usually confined to genitalia or perianal region. These appear as one or more tender papules, becoming pustular and eroding to form non-indurated painful ulcers. Lesions may coalesce and become secondarily infected.
- Secondary lesion in inguinal lymph nodes, usually unilateral. Swollen lymph nodes are painful and may suppurate. Rupture of abscess may leave discharging sinus.
- Chancroid coexists with syphilis in up to 10% of patients.

Laboratory diagnosis
- Microscopy: in 50% of cases possible to demonstrate pleomorphic, Gram-negative rods in exudate from the ulcer edge.
- Culture: *H. ducreyi* has fastidious growth requirements and culture is not available in most routine laboratories.

Treatment
- Tetracycline 500 mg by mouth for at least 10 days. Some strains resistant, especially in South East Asia.
- Co-trimoxazole one tablet (480 mg) four times a day by mouth for at least 7 days.

Prevention

Immediate
- Isolation: wound precautions.
- Early specific treatment.
- Avoid sexual contact until lesions healed.
- Report to health authority or sexually-transmitted disease (STD) clinic.
- Trace sexual contacts; specific treatment whether or not symptoms are present.

Longterm
- Health education to limit spread of STD.
- Early detection and treatment of cases and sexual contacts.

Chlamydial infections

Organisms
Obligate intracellular parasites, in size between bacteria and viruses. Complex form of replication ending in binary fission, forming intracytoplasmic, basophilic inclusions; contain both nucleic acids; sensitive to certain antibacterial antibiotics. Differentiated into two groups sharing a complement-fixing antigen: *Chlamydia trachomatis* group which forms compact, iodine-staining inclusions and *C. psittaci*, which forms diffuse, non-iodine-staining inclusions.

1 *Chlamydia trachomatis*

Epidemiology

Distribution
Infection worldwide, common; causing a range of diseases affecting the eye and genital tract, which vary with the serotype of *C. trachomatis* involved and with environmental conditions.

Serotypes A, B, Ba and C cause trachoma in tropical and subtropical areas; associated with poor living conditions, usually in rural areas; commonest in children; may lead to visual impairment.

Serotypes D to K cause genital infections; in UK over 100 000 cases of non-specific genital infection reported per year (1980–86), about half due to chlamydiae; probably main cause of rise in pelvic inflammatory disease in women (over 20 000 hospital inpatients in 1986). Ophthalmia neonatorum often due to *C. trachomatis*; pneumonitis in infants may occur; inclusion conjunctivitis in older children and adults.

Serotypes L1, L2 and L3 cause lymphogranuloma venereum (LGV); common in tropics, rare in temperate zones; in UK less than 50 reported cases per year 1980–86.

Source
Human: cases or subclinical infection.

Spread
Direct or indirect contact. Eye infection usually spread by hands, from genital secretions of infected persons or by auto-infection, rarely by

water in swimming pools with defective or no disinfection; trachoma may be flyborne; ophthalmia neonatorum and infant pneumonitis by direct contact during birth. Genital infections usually spread by sexual intercourse.

Pathogenesis

Lymphogranuloma venereum
Ill understood. Plasma cell and histiocytic infiltration around primary lesion. Regional lymphatic involvement, often with gumma-like necrosis. Proliferation of fibrous tissue in healing lesions, leading to stricture formation.

Trachoma
Conjunctival lesion with mononuclear cellular infiltration, forms enlarging inflammatory follicles. Later, infiltration and vascularization of cornea, progressing to ulceration.

Clinical features

Genital infection — non-gonococcal urethritis
- *C. trachomatis* isolated from urethra in up to 5% of symptomless men, 20% of men with gonorrhoea and 30−50% of men with non-specific urethritis; isolated from the cervix in up to 60% of women with gonorrhoea.
- Chlamydial urethritis is clinically indistinguishable from gono-coccal, but is milder; also epididymitis.
- Cervicitis, salpingitis, proctitis and diffuse peritonitis (FitzHugh−Curtis syndrome).
- Association with Reiter's syndrome.

Genital infection — LGV
Incubation period is usually 7−15 days but may extend to 5 weeks.
Early lesions:
- Primary lesion consists of small painless papule or ulcer anywhere on genitalia or in rectum; rarely recognized in women. Heals quickly without scarring.
- Regional lymphadenitis follows in few days to weeks. Painful

enlargement of lymph nodes; periadenitis with matting: multiple small abscesses and sinus formation.
● Constitutional symptoms variable: fever, shivering, headache, malaise and arthralgia.
● Most abscesses heal in weeks or months leaving characteristic scarring.
Late lesions:
● Fistulae involving vagina, bladder or bowel.
● Perianal abscess.
● Anorectal stricture in women or homosexual men.
● Lymphatic oedema, especially of vulva or penis.

Eye infections
Incubation period is usually 3–7 days: may range from 1–10 days.
● *Inclusion conjunctivitis in the newborn*: onset of mucopurulent conjunctivitis within 2 weeks of birth. May be unilateral or bilateral. No distinguishing clinical features. Acute stage settles after 2 weeks but the eye may take several months to return to normal. May progress to mild trachoma.
● *Inclusion conjunctivitis in adults*: acute onset of mucopurulent conjunctivitis. Conjunctival follicles and keratitis. Heals slowly over a period of 1–2 years.
● *Trachoma*: persistent or recurrent infection may give rise to chronic keratoconjunctivitis and lead to pannus, scarring of the conjunctivae and ultimate blindness.

Respiratory infections
● Nasopharyngeal infection may be found in otherwise healthy neonates.
● Interstitial pneumonia may develop insidiously within 2–3 months of birth. Follows protracted course and signs may persist for months. Temperature remains normal.

Laboratory diagnosis

Trachoma, urethritis
● *Microscopy*: inclusions demonstrable by Giemsa or immunofluorescent staining of epithelial scrapings; relatively insensitive.

Chlamydial infections: *Chlamydia trachomatis*

Laboratory diagnosis

- *Culture*: appropriate swabs inoculated into irradiated McCoy or Hela cell tissue culture: after 48−72 hours examined by immunofluorescence
- *Serology*: humoral antibody detection by indirect immunofluorescence. Complement fixation test (CFT) less sensitive.

LGV
- *Culture*: not used.
- *Serology*: as above.

Treatment

Genital infections
- Tetracycline 500 mg 6-hourly for 7−21 days.
- Sulphadiazine 5 g in divided doses daily for 5−10 days, or co-trimoxazole two tablets twice daily for 10 days.
- Erythromycin 500 mg 6-hourly for 10−14 days.
- Surgery for fistulae or strictures.

Eye infections
- Oral sulphonamides or tetracycline for adults; course 2−3 weeks.
- Erythromycin or sulphonamides for infants.
- Surgery to correct deformities.

Respiratory infections
- Sulphadimidine 150 mg/kg/day for 2−3 weeks.
- Erythromycin 50 mg/kg/day for 2−3 weeks.

Prevention

Immediate
- Isolation: unnecessary for genital infections; wound precautions for eye infections; respiratory precautions for pneumonitis.
- Early specific treatment.
- Report to health authority or STD clinic. Ophthalmia neonatorum notifiable in UK.
- Trace sexual contacts, surveillance and treatment.

Prevention

Longterm
- Health education to limit spread of STD.
- Prophylactic treatment of neonates exposed to infection with topical tetracycline 1% and oral erythromycin 25–50 mg/kg daily for 3 weeks.
- Maintenance of hygiene in swimming pools.
- Trachoma control programmes in endemic areas by mass treatment with tetracycline eye ointment, usually intermittent treatment twice daily for 6 days every 6 months.

2 *Chlamydia psittaci*

Epidemiology

Distribution
Worldwide infection usually sporadic. Common in persons occupationally exposed to psittacines, such as pet-shop and aviary workers, in whom the disease may be severe; also in those exposed to other birds, such as pigeon keepers, workers in duck- and turkey-processing plants (ornithosis). Milder non-pneumonic respiratory disease described in outbreaks apparently spread from person to person. Reported also in farmers and their families exposed to enzootic abortion in ewes; may cause fetal death and abortion in pregnant women. An important hazard to laboratory workers handling the organism; nosocomial infection has been reported.

Source
Symptomless or sick birds and poultry, ewes with enzootic abortion. Rarely human.

Spread
Airborne: inhalation of dust from faeces or feathers of infected birds; aerosol from infected ewes at lambing, from person to person, from specimens in laboratories. Possibly by direct contact in these cases.

Pathogenesis
Unilateral patchy pulmonary consolidation, presumably at site of

lodgement of inhaled particles. Severe infections uncommon but associated with extensive pneumonia, bloodstream invasion and circulatory collapse.

Clinical features

Incubation period
Commonly about 10 days but may extend from a few days to 4 weeks.

Other features
- Mild attacks resemble influenza.
- Severe attacks begin with an influenza-like illness. During first week the patient may have epistaxis and gastrointestinal disturbance with diarrhoea. High fever with relative bradycardia. Dry cough with minimal chest signs. Evidence of consolidation in second week. Extent of pneumonia on radiological examination out of proportion to the physical signs. ESR (erythrocyte sedimentation rate) tends to be markedly increased.
- Occasional rose-spot rash. Apathy and mental confusion. Myocardial damage.
- Illness subsides after 7–14 days but convalescence may be protracted and radiological clearance takes several weeks.

Laboratory diagnosis

Serology
Complement-fixing antibodies against an antigen shared between *C. psittaci* and other chlamydiae detectable during acute stage of infection. Tests for species-specific antibodies not usually performed.

Culture
Sputum or blood can be inoculated into chick yolk sac or intraperitoneally into mice; serological diagnosis is more common.

Treatment
Chlortetracycline or oxytetracycline 500 mg 6-hourly orally until fever subsides, then 250 mg 6-hourly. Total course 10–14 days.

Prevention

Immediate
- Isolation: respiratory precautions during acute stage.
- Identify contacts possibly exposed to same source of infection for surveillance and treatment if necessary.
- Report to health authority so that source and spread may be investigated; notifiable in some parts of UK.
- In hospitals and laboratories, inform control-of-infection officer.
- Report animal infection to agricultural authority.

Longterm
- Supervision of pet shops to prevent sale of infected birds.
- Restriction on imported psittacines.
- Ventilation and hygiene in poultry-processing plants.
- Pregnant women should be advised not to work with ewes during the lambing season.
- Special care in handling laboratory specimens.

Cholera

Organism
Vibrio cholerae: curved, actively motile, Gram-negative rod. More than 80 O serotypes; type O1 responsible for epidemic cholera. Further differentiation of type O1 possible into inaba and ogawa serotypes and El Tor biotype. Serotypes O2, O3, etc. referred to variously as 'non-cholera vibrios' or *V. cholerae* non-O1. Some of the strains cause diarrhoea (less severe than O1 strains), others are non-pathogens.

Epidemiology

Distribution
Pandemic of cholera, El Tor biotype, beginning in Indonesia 1961 and reaching Europe 1970. In UK 51 cases and two deaths, 1970−87, all imported; no spread of disease. Sporadic cases of diarrhoea, sometimes outbreaks, caused by non-cholera vibrios (non-O1 *V. cholerae* and atypical *V. cholerae* O1); but these organisms do not have same epidemic potential as *V. cholerae* O1 and do not require same control measures.

Source
Human case or, less commonly, carrier. There may be environmental reservoirs of non-culturable organisms.

Spread
Faecal contamination of water, sometimes food; shellfish harvested from sewage polluted waters. Person-to-person spread uncommon.

Pathogenesis
V. cholerae are not invasive organisms but produce a potent enterotoxin which, in the severely affected patient, causes the loss of large volumes of fluid and electrolytes from mucosal cells of the lower gastrointestinal tract. Less severe symptoms, or even subclinical infections, are more common in El Tor infections than in classical cholera and in the previously healthy and well-nourished.

Clinical features

Incubation
Usually 1–3 days; up to 5 days.

Mild
Resembles gastroenteritis; usually caused by El Tor biotype.

Severe
Onset abrupt; diarrhoea followed by vomiting; loss of large volumes of colourless liquid leads to severe dehydration, circulatory and renal failure; stools do not contain blood; diarrhoea lessens after 2–12 hours; recovery slow.

Laboratory diagnosis

Microscopy
Where disease is epidemic, presumptive diagnosis of clinically recognized case by microscopy of peptone-water suspension of 'rice-water' stool; actively motile, comma-shaped organisms seen.

Culture
Typical colonies on appropriate selective media; identified by biochemical and serological tests. In countries where cholera is not endemic and where facilities exist, identification should be confirmed by reference laboratory.

Treatment
- Water and electrolyte replacement.
- Tetracycline 500 mg 6-hourly for 48 hours.
- Chloramphenicol 500 mg 6-hourly for resistant strains.

Prevention

Immediate
- Isolation: enteric precautions.
- Exclude from food handling until three consecutive negative faecal specimens at intervals of not less than 48 hours.

Cholera

<u>Prevention</u>

- Report to health authority; notifiable in UK.
- Identify household contacts and those exposed to same source of infection; bacteriological screening; surveillance for 5 days after contact; consider tetracycline prophylaxis.
- Exclude contacts from food handling, as above.
- Immunization not appropriate.

Longterm
- Hygienic disposal of sewage.
- Purification of water supplies.
- Hygienic food production, especially shellfish.
- Immunization (see p. 360).

Colitis

1 Haemorrhagic

Organism
Verotoxin-producing strains of *Escherichia coli*, most commonly O157 H7.

Epidemiology

Distribution
First reported in USA in 1982. Outbreaks and sporadic cases since in North America, Japan, UK. Uncommon; affects all age groups; in UK seasonal peak in July.

Source
Probably zoonosis; bovine. Possibly human.

Spread
Foodborne, meat products often implicated in outbreaks; milkborne. Person to person in families; also outbreaks reported in nurseries and old peoples' homes.

Pathogenesis
● Verotoxin indistinguishable from *Shigella dysenteriae* toxin by Ouchterlony immunodiffusion; also neutralized by rabbit *Sh. dysenteriae* antitoxin; probably acts similarly.
● Oedema, inflammation and haemorrhage of ascending and transverse colon demonstrable.

Clinical features
● Acute bloody diarrhoea.
● Little or no fever.

Laboratory diagnosis
Characterization of faecal strains of *E. coli* unlikely to be performed in routine laboratories. Detection of verotoxin requires facilities of specialist laboratory. Verotoxin-producing strains usually fail to ferment sorbitol.

Treatment
- Clear fluids followed by light low-residue diet.
- Antibiotics not indicated.

Prevention

Immediate
- Isolation: enteric precautions.
- Exclude from food handling until clinically well.
- Report to health authority so that epidemiological investigation may be undertaken.
- Contacts: no action.

Longterm
- None.

2 Necrotizing enterocolitis in infants

Organism
Aetiology unproven but intestinal anaerobes, particularly clostridia, likely to contribute to disease process.

Epidemiology

Distribution
Rare neonatal disease; appears in clusters in hospital.

Source
May be associated with injury to mucosa, and bacterial infection.

Spread
Not known.

Pathogenesis
Not proven, probably multifactorial. Possibly temporary anoxia, or other trauma of bowel permits invasion of epithelium by gas-producing organisms derived from intestinal flora.

Clinical features
- Usually within the first 3 weeks of life with peak incidence 3−10 days.
- Vomiting and bloody diarrhoea.
- Abdominal distension; ileus.
- Plain X-ray of abdomen may show multiple dilated loops of bowel, intramural gas and gas in portal vein.
- Perforation may occur.
- Healing may be complicated by stricture.

Laboratory diagnosis
Usually not attempted but important to exclude recognized infections.

Treatment
- Metronidazole 7.5 mg/kg 8-hourly i.v.
- Reintroduce feeding cautiously, preferably using human milk.

Prevention

Immediate
- Isolation: enteric precautions.
- Inform hospital control-of-infection officer.
- Contacts: no action.

Longterm
- None.

3 Pseudomembranous

Organism
Clostridium difficile: anaerobic, spore-bearing, Gram-positive rod. Probably ubiquitous; possibly a gastrointestinal commensal. Difficult to isolate from a mixed bacterial flora, except with selective media. Non-toxigenic and toxin-producing strains recognized. Toxin cell-necrotizing; cross-antigenicity with *Cl. sordelli* toxin.

Epidemiology

Distribution
Uncommon disease; usually associated with antibiotic therapy, particularly with clindamycin, and often after surgery. Wide variation in incidence; outbreaks in hospitals reported.

Source
Human: cases or carriers.

Spread
Often endogenous, but person to person by faecal−oral route may occur.

Pathogenesis
● Overgrowth of *Cl. difficile* associated with antibiotic-induced interference with intestinal commensals. Factors controlling toxigenicity not understood.
● Toxin apparently responsible for foci of degeneration in epithelium and mucosal glands; superimposed pseudomembrane composed of cellular debris, polymorphs, mucin and fibrin.
● High levels of faecal toxin not necessarily associated with severe disease; duration to exposure to toxin possibly of greater importance.

Clinical features
● Commonly develops within 10 days of starting antibiotic, but may appear 2−3 weeks after completing treatment.
● Fever, abdominal pain and diarrhoea. Stools watery but seldom contain blood.
● Abdominal distension troublesome in severe cases.
● Clinical examination may suggest perforation or formation of abscess.
● Polymorphonuclear leucocytosis; hypoproteinaemia.
● Sigmoidoscopy reveals areas of oedematous congested mucosa with greyish-white plaques of pseudomembrane. Relatively normal mucosa between affected areas in mild cases; confluent lesions in severe attacks.

41

Laboratory diagnosis
- Toxin detectable in filtered faecal suspension in wide range of tissue cultures. Amount of toxin can be estimated by titration, and cytotoxicity neutralized by *Cl. sordelli* antitoxin. Also detectable by counterimmunoelectrophoresis.
- Usually possible to isolate *Cl. difficile* from faeces using appropriate media, but not pathognomonic of disease.

Treatment
- Stop existing antibiotic therapy.
- Replace water and electrolytes. Chemotherapy unnecessary in mild attack.
- Vancomycin 125−500 mg four times a day by mouth for 5−10 days, when attack is severe. Repeat course if necessary.
- Metronidazole often effective and cheaper alternative.
- Corticosteroids sometimes beneficial in severe attack.
- Colectomy may be necessary in overwhelming attack.

Prevention

Immediate
- Isolation: enteric precautions.
- Inform hospital control-of-infection officer.
- Contacts: no action.

Longterm
- Discretion in used of antibiotics, especially clindamycin.
- Hygiene in wards, especially in care of bedpans and commodes.

Congenital and neonatal infections

Organism/disease	Epidemiology	Prevention
Chickenpox (p. 321)	Congenital malformations of various types reported after infection in first trimester.	None
	Neonatal chickenpox rare; infection from non-immune mother with onset of chickenpox within 6 days before birth or during neonatal period, or from other source. Infant zoster has been described	Zoster immunoglobulin may attenuate disease in neonate; recommended for neonates exposed within 4 weeks of birth (p. 324)
Cytomegalovirus (p. 52)	Congenital, following primary infection or reactivation in pregnancy. About 25% infants symptomatic often with severe disease; around 10% of asymptomatic develop disease later.	None; exclusion of pregnant women from working in nurseries and from handling specimens in laboratories is not justified
	Neonatal infection common, especially in nurseries, usually asymptomatic	None
Gram-negative bacteria, including salmonellae (p. 246)	Neonatal infections, giving rise to bacteraemia and meningitis, especially in premature babies, derived from mother's genital tract or perineum, or by faecal−oral spread in hospital infant units	Faecal examination of mothers on admission to maternity units and isolation until shown to be free of salmonellae, has been suggested
Group B streptococci (p. 285)	Neonatal infection derived from genital tract	Bacteriological screening and chemoprophylaxis

Organism/disease/epidemiology/prevention

Organism/disease	Epidemiology	Prevention
	of mother in early neonatal septicaemia (about 5–25% of women infected). Late neonatal meningitis may be due to person-to-person spread	of positive mothers, and chemoprophylaxis of 'high-risk' infants has been suggested
Hepatitis B (p. 120)	Perinatal infection from carrier mother, especially HBeAg carrier, or maternal infection in late pregnancy or puerperium. Carrier rates high in some ethnic groups. Infected infants likely to become carriers and to develop chronic liver disease, including primary hepatic carcinoma	Infants of mothers with hepatitis B during last trimester or early puerperium, and of carrier mothers: hepatitis B immunoglobulin within 24 hours after birth or exposure, and hepatitis B vaccine (p. 127)
Herpes simplex (p. 129)	Congenital infections rare. Perinatal infections from lesions of birth canal. Rarely case-to-case spread in neonatal nurseries	Isolation: secretion precautions of infants. Caesarean section has been recommended when lesions of birth canal within 2 weeks of expected date of delivery. Antiviral drugs may be of value in prophylaxis
HIV infection (p. 133)	Infection may occur *in utero*, from blood or cervical secretions during birth, or from breast milk during neonatal period. Risk of infection not yet known but may be as high as	Advice to infected and 'high-risk' women against pregnancy. Therapeutic abortion should be considered

Congenital and neonatal infections

Organism/disease/epidemiology/prevention

Organism/disease	Epidemiology	Prevention
	65% in mothers who have previously transmitted HIV infection	
Listeriosis (p. 157)	Abortion. Neonatal septicaemia and meningitis; early due to intrauterine infection, late to infection from mother's genital tract or environment	Pregnant women should avoid contact with animal sources of infection, such as aborting farm animals. Ampicillin prophylaxis has been suggested for newborn infants of infected mothers
Parvovirus (B19) infection (p. 205)	Abortion may follow infection (erythema infectiosum) in pregnancy. Hydrops foetalis has been reported but malformations not described	None
Rubella (p. 241)	Maternal infection in first trimester is followed by congenital rubella syndrome in about 25% of infants; defects in almost all infants of mothers infected in first 7 weeks of pregnancy, usually severe affecting heart, eye and CNS; defects not recorded following infections after 17 weeks of pregnancy	Rubella immunization before pregnancy (p. 358). Therapeutic abortion following infection in pregnancy
Syphilis (p. 299)	Congenital syphilis due to transplacental infection from mother with untreated early syphilis	Antenatal serological screening and treatment of positive mothers

Congenital and neonatal infections

Organism/disease/epidemiology/prevention

Organism/disease	Epidemiology	Prevention
Toxoplasmosis (p. 295)	Congenital infection occurs in about 40% of infants of mothers primarily infected in pregnancy, most of the infected infants develop disease. Lowest risk of transmission but severest disease in early pregnancy. Usually no risk in subsequent pregnancies, except in immunocompromised mothers	Avoid contact during pregnancy with likely sources of infection: raw or undercooked meat, garden soil, cat faeces and litter Therapeutic abortion

Conjunctivitis

General features

Conjunctivitis is a component of many systemic infections. e.g. measles, rubella, leptospirosis, tularaemia, Reiter's disease. It may follow exposure to chemicals or toxins, or be an allergic manifestation. Other diseases of the eye, such as glaucoma, may present with pain, lachrymation and hyperaemia. Conjunctivitis *per se* is caused by a wide variety of micro-organisms, and in addition there are several specific syndromes.

The normal eye has several defences against infection:

- The unhampered flow of lachrymal secretions.
- Antibacterial activity of tears (salinity and lysozyme).
- Mechanical wiping by the eyelids.

The eye of the neonate is more readily infected because:

- The lachrymal ducts may not be patent.
- There may be qualitative deficiencies in the tears.
- There may be exposure to potential pathogens during birth.

1 Specific syndromes

Organisms

- Adenoviruses types 3, 4, 7, 8.
- ECHOvirus type 70.
- *Chlamydia trachomatis*.
- *Listeria monocytogenes*.
- *Haemophilus aegyptius*.
- Acanthamoeba: free-living amoebae.

Clinical syndromes

Acute follicular conjunctivitis

- *C. trachomatis* (genital strain).
- Spread by direct or indirect contact.
- Lower eyelid more affected than upper; superficial punctate keratitis.
- Prevention: personal hygiene; hygiene of swimming pools.

Clinical syndromes

Acute haemorrhagic conjunctivitis
- Enterovirus 70 first reported in Far East in 1970 and since reported in many parts of the world. Also associated with Coxsackie virus A24.
- Spreads readily by direct or indirect contact with eye discharges, especially where hygiene standards are low.
- Sudden onset of severe bilateral conjunctivitis with subconjunctival haemorrhages. Transient slight keratitis. Recovery 1–2 weeks.
- Neurological complication: acute radiculomyelopathy.

Epidemic keratoconjunctivitis
- Adenovirus types 3, 7, 8.
- Worldwide; respiratory spread; also by direct or indirect contact, e.g. by ophthalmic instruments. Associated with eye injury in shipyard workers (shipyard eye) and in other occupations.
- Scanty exudate; keratitis.
- Prevention: avoid overcrowding; personal hygiene; ensure sterility of instruments.

Pharyngoconjunctival fever
- Adenovirus types 3, 4 and others.
- History of swimming common.
- Associated with pharyngitis (p. 238).

Listeriosis
- *Listeria monocytogenes* (p. 157).
- Oculoglandular: purulent discharge from eyes; inflammation of salivary glands progressing to suppuration.
- Purulent conjunctivitis in poultry workers.

Brazilian purpuric fever
- *Haemophilus aegyptius*.
- Purulent conjunctivitis.
- Reported in Brazil in 1984 with ensuing generalized illness, fever and purpura.
- Affects children; high fatality rate reported in recognized cases.

Acanthamoeba infection
- Associated with the wearing of contact lenses and the use of non-sterile cleaning solution.
- Invasion of cornea causing keratitis.

2 Non-specific syndromes

Clinical syndromes

Acute serous
Mucosal congestion, diffuse conjunctival swelling, watery discharge. Aetiological agents:
- Newcastle virus: causes respiratory disease in poultry; human infection is confined to persons in close contact with infected flocks or working in poultry-processing plants. Unilateral conjunctivitis common.
- Adenovirus.
- Herpes simplex virus: may be recurrent.

Acute catarrhal and purulent
Considerable overlap between two syndromes. Clinical features of catarrhal infection: moderate congestion with mucus discharge. Purulent infection: severe congestion with purulent discharge; may also have corneal involvement. Persistent or recurrent infection associated with blockage of nasolachrymal duct. Aetiological agents include:
- *Neisseria gonorrhoeae**: ophthalmia neonatorum from infected birth canal; maternal infection should be treated during pregnancy; if inadequately treated, antibiotic eyedrops should be used prophylactically at birth.
- *Staph. aureus* and *Staph. epidermidis.**
- *Strep. pneumoniae.*
- *Strep. pyogenes.*
- *H. influenzae.*
- Enterobacteria.*

* Of especial importance in neonates and infants.

Clinical syndromes

- *Pseudomonas aeruginosa*:* may be derived from contaminated eyedrops and contaminated water in humidifiers of ventilating systems. Ensure strict sterility of these substances.
- *C. trachomatis*:* ophthalmia neonatorum — see above.
- Herpes simplex virus.

Acute membranous
- Diphtheritic conjunctivitis may occur as part of a generalized infection or as an isolated manifestation.
- May also be caused by severe infection with *Strep. pyogenes.*
- Reddened oedematous conjunctiva with membrane formation especially on palpebral surface.

Subacute or chronic
Angular:
- *Moraxella lacunata*.
- Infrequently reported, causes outbreaks in children in enclosed communities, spread by direct and indirect contact.
- Gradual onset and slow evolution. Pain out of proportion to inflammation. Vascular engorgement at angles of conjunctival sac.
Follicular:
- Worldwide infection caused by *C. trachomatis*.
- Spread by direct or indirect contact.
- Trachoma in tropics; inclusion conjunctivitis in temperate zones (p. 30).

Laboratory diagnosis
- Specimens for bacterial culture should be taken with a small sterile loop from conjunctival secretions. Blood agar and chocolate agar plates should be inoculated at the patient's side (lysozyme may destroy microorganisms if there is any delay in culturing). If immediate culture is impossible then a fine swab must be used and placed in bacterial transport medium without delay.
- Chlamydial and virus specimens, taken with fine swabs, are immediately placed in the appropriate transport media and refrigerated (or stored at -70°C if culture will be delayed).

* Of especial importance in neonates and infants.

Conjunctivitis: Non-specific syndromes

Laboratory diagnosis

- Chlamydial infections may be recognized by demonstrating intra-cytoplasmic inclusions in conjunctival scrapings stained with iodine or Giemsa's stain.
- In pharyngoconjunctival fever adenovirus may be isolated from the pharynx or faeces, and humoral antibodies demonstrated.

Treatment

- Most viral forms of conjunctivitis will subside spontaneously within 2−3 weeks and do not require specific therapy.
- Herpes simplex conjunctivitis responds to treatment with acyclovir or adenine arabinoside or idoxuridine applied locally.
- Purulent conjunctivitis: culture and determine sensitivity of organism and treat accordingly. Topical antibiotics include chloramphenicol, framycetin, gentamicin, neomycin and polymyxin B.
- Gonococcal conjunctivitis: benzylpenicillin or procaine penicillin i.m. for 4−7 days or eyedrops containing chloramphenicol every 10 minutes for the first 30 minutes, then hourly until the infection responds, then less frequently.
- Trachoma: sulphadimidine, sulphadiazine or tetracycline by mouth. Local treatment using chlortetracycline ointment is less effective.
- Inclusion conjunctivitis: tetracycline orally or locally for 2−3 weeks.
- Corticosteroid drops must be used with caution and are not indicated unless there is severe keratitis causing reduction in vision.

Cytomegalovirus infection

Organism
One of the herpes group of DNA viruses. Human strains can be propagated on human fibroblast and myometrial cells but animal strains
rarely grow on human cells.

Epidemiology

Distribution
Worldwide, very common, usually symptomless. Congenital infection
in 0.5−2% of live births due to primary infection in pregnancy or less
commonly to reactivation of virus in immune mothers; up to 25%
babies symptomatic, sometimes severe, fatal disease; about 10%
asymptomatic babies develop manifestations later, such as neuro-
sensory hearing loss. Perinatal and childhood infections nearly
always asymptomatic. Adult infections may cause mononucleosis
and sometimes hepatitis. Infection common and often disseminated
in transplant recipients and in other immunosuppressed patients; a
serious manifestation of Aids.

Source
Human: virus excreted in urine and saliva for long periods, particularly after infection in infancy.

Spread
Transplacental: from infected cervix during birth; breast milk; close
contact in children and young adults, such as kissing; sexual intercourse; transfusion of fresh blood; organ transplant.

Pathogenesis

Histological picture
Enlarged cells containing intranuclear (owl eye) and cytoplasmic
inclusions widely disseminated throughout body.

Kidneys
Interstitial nephritis.

Cytomegalovirus infection

Lungs
Pneumonitis with focal infiltration by mononuclear cells.

Brain
Necrotic granulomatous lesions and extensive calcification.

Clinical features

Congenital
- *Asymptomatic*: 75% or more.
- *Acute fulminating*: onset within 48 hours of birth; jaundice, hepatosplenomegaly, thrombocytopenic purpura and anaemia. Most severely affected survivors show evidence of damage to CNS.
- *Malformations*: may be found in heart, gastrointestinal tract, brain and kidneys. Microcephaly a common finding.

Postnatal
- *Children*: most infections not recognized; occasionally evidence of liver damage; general involvement rare; CNS not affected.
- *Adults*: usually subclinical; cytomegalovirus mononucleosis as natural event and as post-transfusion syndrome 2–7 months after fresh-blood transfusion, manifesting with prolonged fever, non-icteric hepatitis, a high proportion of atypical mononuclear cells in the peripheral blood and negative Paul–Bunnell or Monospot test; pneumonitis with distinctive nodular shadows found in immunocompromised patients.

Important cause of prolonged fever in transplant patients. Chorioretinitis is major late manifestation in transplant patients (see also Aids, p. 136).

Laboratory diagnosis
- *Culture*: urine, throat swab, bronchiolar lavage in fibroblast cell lines.
- *Direct microscopy of urine*: typical large cells with intranuclear inclusions; culture more sensitive.
- *Serology*: Specific IgM antibodies detectable in current or recent infections. Rapid methods for virus antigen detection available in specialist laboratories.

Treatment
- Antiviral agents ineffective. Symptomatic treatment for most cases.
- Transfusion of packed red cells and of platelet-rich plasma in fulminating cases.

Prevention

Immediate
- Isolation: wound precautions.
- Contacts: no action.

Longterm
- Exclusion of women in childbearing years from working in nurseries or handling specimens in laboratories has been suggested because of high prevalence of infection in infants and high infection rates of urine specimens but is not justified. Studies have demonstrated that the risk of infection in these circumstances is minimal. Strict standards of hygiene, particularly handwashing, should be maintained.
- Blood transfusion: seronegative blood for seronegative recipients who are immunosuppressed.
- Organ donation: matching so that seronegative donor organs are given to seronegative recipients.

Dengue

Organisms
Dengue virus: RNA virus, approximately 17−25 nm in diameter; four serotypes; one of the arboviruses (group B). Several distinct viruses, including chikungunya virus, can cause a similar clinical picture.

Epidemiology

Distribution
Common in tropics and subtropics, especially Caribbean and South East Asia. Haemorrhagic disease, mainly in children, may follow sensitization by previous recent infection with different virus serotype, most frequent in India, South East Asia and Pacific (see p. 326).

Source
Human. Possibly monkeys.

Spread
Mosquitoes, *Aedes* spp. usually *A. aegypti*.

Pathogenesis
The disease centres upon small blood vessels, in which there is endo-thelial swelling, perivascular oedema and mononuclear infiltration. The varying severity of infection may be due to different host suscep-tibility, dosage effect or some alteration in virulence of the virus.

Clinical features

Incubation period
Usually 5−9 days.

Onset
Sudden with fever, chills, severe headache, retro-orbital pain, dis-tressing joint and muscle pains (breakbone fever) progressing to intense prostration. Some have biphasic 'saddle-back' pattern of fever.

Other features
Lymphadenopathy, neutropenia. Rashes days 3—5: maculopapular,
erythematous or petechial.

Course
Usually 5—7 days.

Haemorrhagic dengue
Minor febrile illness for 2—4 days followed by sudden deterioration
with hepatomegaly, disseminated intravascular coagulation (DIC) and
hypovolaemic shock. Mortality of 5—10%.

Laboratory diagnosis
• Precise diagnosis only by isolation of virus, but this is rarely
practicable.
• Serology is of limited value in an acute episode as antibody persists for long periods after a primary infection, and may cross-react
with other arboviruses.

Treatment
• Symptomatic: analgesics, bedrest.
• Plasma infusion for shock.

Prevention

Immediate
Report outbreaks to health authority to enable identification of localities affected and to implement emergency mosquito control.

Longterm
Mosquito control; protection against mosquitoes.

Diphtheria

Organisms

Corynebacterium diphtheriae: important pathogen in a genus of aerobic, Gram-positive rods comprising usually less virulent species, *C. ulcerans and C. haemolyticum*, and commensals (diphtheroids). Virulent strains produce a polypeptide exotoxin; non-toxigenic strains cause local infection only.

Epidemiology

Distribution
Worldwide, mainly children, rare in countries with effective childhood immunization programmes. In UK, average 4 cases per year 1980–87, most in unimmunized children, often associated with imported infection.

Source
Nose or throat of human case or carrier. In tropics infected skin lesions common. *C. ulcerans*, cattle.

Spread
Close contact with infected secretions. Fomites rarely play a part. *C. ulcerans*, milkborne.

Pathogenesis
- *C. diphtheriae* causes superficial infection.
- Cellular damage results in formation of a pseudomembrane.
- Toxin diffuses widely in circulation and inhibits host cell function by interfering with protein synthesis.

Clinical features

Incubation period
Usually 1–3 days.

Onset
Insidious with listlessness, low-grade fever or subnormal temperature, tachycardia. Seldom pain.

Course
Depends on site of infection.

Site	Local lesion	Toxicity
Respiratory		
Nasal	Offensive bloodstained watery discharge; excoriation round nostrils	Seldom toxic
Tonsillar	Membrane confined to tonsils; edge well-demarcated	Moderate toxicity
Nasopharyngeal	Extensive membrane; marked oedema; spreading edge difficult to define	Extreme toxaemia; subnormal temperature; hypotension; cardiac failure
Laryngeal	Progressive obstruction	Moderate toxaemia
Tracheobronchial	Severe obstruction not relieved by tracheostomy or intubation; bronchopneumonia	Severe toxaemia
Non-respiratory		
Wounds; skin lesions; eye; genital tract	Easily overlooked; consider in gravely ill; indolent wounds with offensive discharge; membranous conjunctivitis	Toxicity very variable

Complications
● Myocarditis appears about days 8–10 with tachycardia and arrhythmia. Death from cardiac arrest or circulatory failure commonly occurs about the 15th day. In survivors, cardiac function is restored to normal.
● Neuropathy involves motor nerves and appears sequentially. Palatal paresis about days 14–21; ocular paresis before day 28;

paralysis of muscles of larynx, pharynx or respiration between days 35 and 42; paralysis of limbs as late as day 70. Ultimate recovery is assured.

Laboratory diagnosis
- Clinical diagnosis of prime importance with confirmation by laboratory.
- Microscopy of stained film from site of infection is inadequate to differentiate *C. diphtheriae* from commensals.
- Culture of swabs from nose and throat or other lesions on routine and selective media. Colonies identified biochemically.
- Toxigenicity of strains examined by immunodiffusion (Elek method) or by guinea pig inoculation. Differentiation into gravis, intermedius and mitis strains is not a reliable indicator of toxigenicity.

Treatment
- Immediate antitoxin (see pp. 364−5):
Nasal diphtheria, 8000 units i.m.
Tonsillar and laryngeal, 30 000−40 000 units i.m.
Severe tonsillar, 60 000 units, half i.m., half i.v.
Nasopharyngeal, 100 000−120 000 units, half i.m., half i.v.
- Isolation and bedrest.
- Penicillin or erythromycin to eradicate organism.

Prevention

Immediate
- Isolation: respiratory/wound precautions.
- Cases and carriers: continue isolation until three negative nose and throat swabs at 2−3 day intervals, the first at least 5 days after completion of antibiotic therapy.
- Report to health authority. Notifiable in UK and most countries.
- Search for source of infection by identifying missed cases, including cutaneous diphtheria.
- Identify close contacts, that is persons exposed to secretions of case or carrier and usually limited to persons in same household or school class; take nose and throat swabs for culture.

Diphtheria

Prevention

- Prophylaxis for contacts

Age	History of primary immunization		
	Complete course with or without reinforcing dose		None or incomplete or not known
	<6 months before	6+ months before	
<10 years	None	Dip/Vac/Ads or DT/Vac/Ads 0.5 ml i.m.	Dip/Vac/Ads or DT/Vac/Ads 0.5 ml i.m. plus antibiotics*
10+ years	None	Dip/Vac/Ads for adults 0.5 ml i.m.	Dip/Vac/Ads for adults 0.5 ml i.m. plus antibiotics*

* Complete primary immunization by giving two further doses at intervals of 1 month. Erythromycin 125–250 mg orally 6-hourly for 7 days or benzathine penicillin 916 mg i.m. if necessary for compliance.

- Surveillance of contacts: daily for 7 days to detect clinical diphtheria.
- Clearance of contacts: minimum of two negative nose and throat swabs at least 24 hours apart, beginning at least 7 days after contact with case or carrier, at least 5 days after completion of any chemotherapy.
- Persons who are not close contacts: nose and throat swabs and prophylaxis unnecessary; such action may delay detection of cases and carriers among contacts at real risk.
- Carriers of non-toxigenic strains of C. diphtheriae: control measures not necessary.

Longterm
- Routine immunization in infants and high-risk adults (p. 356).

Dysentery

1 Amoebic

Organism

Entamoeba histolytica: protozoan existing as a cyst and as a vegetative (trophozoite) form 10–40 μm in diameter, the larger trophozoites being found in active infections. Encysting does not take place in tissues but may in faeces; transmission is by the cyst.

Epidemiology

Distribution
Worldwide; widespread in areas of poor sanitation particularly in the tropics; common in promiscuous homosexual men and in patients in mental hospitals; infection frequently symptomless. About 100 hospitalized cases a year in UK 1980–87.

Source
Human faeces, usually from chronic case or symptomless excreter of cysts; acute case not commonly a source.

Spread
Faecal–oral route; waterborne; foodborne from raw vegetables contaminated with polluted water or from food contaminated by infected food handler or by flies. Sexual contact in homosexuals.

Pathogenesis

Amoebic dysentery affects the caecum and colon. Initially lesions are confined to the mucosa, tending to spread laterally, then extending via small vessels into the submucosa where narrow-necked lesions are formed. Spread of infection occurs within the intestinal tract or via the portal circulation to the liver (amoebic abscess) and, by local extension or via the bloodstream, to the lungs and occasionally other sites, such as the brain.

Clinical features

- Incubation period uncertain: 1–2 weeks or longer.
- Onset insidious. Usually apyrexial.
- Toxic manifestations absent.

Clinical features

- Vomiting not a feature.
- Diarrhoea mild, occasionally severe.
- Abdominal pain and tenesmus uncommon.
- Stools semiformed or bloodstained mucus. Very offensive; resemble anchovy sauce. Less numerous and have greater bulk than those in bacillary dysentery.
- Sigmoidoscopy reveals ulcers.
- Duration a few days to a few weeks. Remission followed by relapse.
- Complications:
Local: haemorrhage, perforation, peritonitis, amoeboma.
Metastatic: abscess liver, lung or brain.

Laboratory diagnosis

Microscopy
Must be carried out on freshly passed faeces; mucoid or blood·stained portions are examined for the larger trophozoites; red blood cells (RBCs) should be visible within amoebae. Demonstration of cysts or small trophozoites is not diagnostic of acute infection; persistence is common. Cysts of non-pathogenic amoebae are common but usually less than 10 μm in diameter; the distinction is readily made with experience. RBCs present in rouleaux formation, macrophages scarce or absent, few pus cells, Charcot−Leyden crystals.

Serology
Detection of humoral antibodies by immunofluorescence (IF) and cellulose-acetate precipitation (CAP) is particularly useful in the differential diagnosis of amoebic liver abscess. Antibodies detected in more than 90% of patients with invasive amoebiasis and about 75% of patients with amoebic dysentery. CAP becomes positive after 10−14 days and reverts to negative after treatment.

Treatment

Acute dysentery
- Metronidazole 800 mg three times a day by mouth for 10 days; *or*
- Metronidazole 800 mg three times a day by mouth for 5 days

Treatment

---

followed by diloxanide fuorate 500 mg three times a day by mouth for 10 days.
- Re-examine stools after 1 month.

Cyst carriers
- Treatment seldom necessary. Many cysts non-pathogenic. Most disappear within a few weeks or months.
- Treat if serology is positive or person is a food handler.
- Diloxanide fuorate drug of choice: 500 mg three times a day for 10 days.

Liver abscess
- Aspiration of large abscess shortens illness.
- Metronidazole 400 mg three times a day by mouth for 5–10 days.
- Chloroquine, 600 mg of base by mouth daily for 5 days followed by 300 mg daily for 14–21 days, is less effective.
- Diloxanide as above on completion of metronidazole or chloroquine.

Prevention

Immediate
- Isolation: enteric precautions.
- Prompt treatment with metronidazole.
- Report to health authority. Dysentery notifiable in UK.
- Contacts: epidemiological investigation and faecal examination of household contacts and other persons possibly exposed to infection in order to identify source and spread. Treatment of contacts found to be infected (see above).
- Exclude cases and cyst excreters from food handling until treatment completed and three negative faeces specimens examined for cysts.

Longterm
- Hygienic sewage disposal.
- Purification of water supplies.
- Education in food hygiene and personal hygiene.
- Fly control.

2 Bacillary

Organism

Non-motile, Gram-negative bacilli belonging to the genus *Shigella*. Several species, including *Sh. sonnei, Sh. flexneri, Sh. boydii, Sh. dysenteriae I (shigae), Sh. dysenteriae II (schmitzii)*. Only one, *Sh. dysenteriae I*, produces an exotoxin and it is noteworthy that this organism is associated with the severest attacks. *Sh. sonnei* generally produces mild illness.

Epidemiology

Distribution

Worldwide; common in children; outbreaks in nurseries, primary schools, mental hospitals and in circumstances of overcrowding and poor hygiene. *Sh. sonnei* causes mild childhood disease in Europe, North America, Australasia; in UK average about 5000 cases reported annually, 1980−87. *Sh. flexneri*, about 400 cases per year in UK 1980−87, usually adults, frequent in patients in mental institutions; imported infections common. *Sh. boydii* and *Sh. dysenteriae* rare in UK and usually imported, may cause severe disease; common in Asia, Africa and South America where extensive waterborne and foodborne outbreaks have been reported.

Source

Human faeces during acute infection; less commonly symptomless excreters. May infect monkeys but not a significant source.

Spread

Faecal−oral route in children and under poor conditions of hygiene. Waterborne; milkborne; foodborne; transmitted by flies.

Pathogenesis

Invasion of villi of intestinal mucosa, causing necrosis and haemorrhage. Ulcers usually heal leaving normal mucosa. In severest cases fibrosis may lead to stenosis. *Sh. dysenteriae I* produces an exotoxin which adds to local pathogenicity. Shigellae, especially *Sh. dysenteriae*, may occasionally invade the bloodstream.

Clinical features
- Incubation: 10 hours to 7 days, usually 2−3 days.
- Onset abrupt with fever.
- Toxic manifestations include headache, delirium, meningismus, convulsions in children.
- Vomiting is common in the early stage.
- Diarrhoea is a major feature.
- Stools: watery with mucus, or numerous scanty motions consisting of bright red viscid mucus (red-currant jelly).
- Abdominal pain; general soreness and sharp gripes. Tenesmus common.
- Microscopy: numerous pus cells and macrophages.
- Duration: few days to 2−3 weeks.
- Complications:
  Local: irritable colon, fibrosis, stenosis.
  Allergic: arthritis, iritis.

Laboratory diagnosis
- *Culture*: of faeces (rectal swabs less satisfactory). Identification of species by biochemical and serological reactions.
- *Serology*: examination of sera for humoral antibodies unhelpful.

Treatment

Mild attack
- Clear fluids by mouth followed by light low-residue diet.
- Antidiarrhoeal drugs, such as codeine, diphenoxylate and loperamide, are of secondary importance and should be used with caution, especially in children and the elderly.

Severe attack
- Maintain fluid balance by i.v. infusion.
- Antibiotic according to sensitivity of organism. Marked regional variation.

Allergic complications
- Aspirin or non-steroidal anti-inflammatory drug for mild arthritis.
- Injection of corticosteroid into joint may be required in severe or prolonged bout.

Treatment

• Local treatment with corticosteroid and atropine eyedrops for iritis. Seek expert advice.

Prevention

Immediate
• Isolation: enteric precautions.
• Report to health authority; notifiable in UK.
• Epidemiological investigation of possible related cases to determine source and spread.
• Contacts: bacteriological screening of well contacts not justified unless food handlers, health-care workers, or there are other circumstances which increase the risk of spread.
• Clearance: food handlers, health-care or nursery staff, children under 5 years of age, and adults with poor standards of hygiene, who pose a special risk of spread, should be excluded from work or school until three consecutive negative faecal specimens have been obtained at intervals of at least 24 hours. Others need not be excluded when asymptomatic.

Longterm
• Hygienic disposal of sewage.
• Purification of water supplies.
• Education to prevent faecal−oral spread, especially in infant and nursery schools.
• Food hygiene; personal hygiene of food handlers; fly control.

3 Schistosomal

Organisms
The trematodes (flukes) *Schistosoma mansoni* and *S. japonicum*.

Epidemiology

Distribution
S. mansoni is located in tropical Africa, the Nile delta and northern South America; *S. japonicum* is located in China, southern Japan and the Philippines.

Dysentery: Schistosomal

Source
S. mansoni human; S. japonicum human and various animals.
Eggs may be excreted in faeces for many years. Intermediate host —
various species of water snail.

Spread
Water containing cercariae (free swimming larvae) which have developed in water snails. The cercariae penetrate the skin of persons
entering the water. Not transmissible from person to person.

Pathogenesis
Both S. mansoni and S. japonicum live in the portal veins, especially
in the tributaries of the inferior mesenteric vein adjacent to the
distal colon. Eggs produced by the worms cause an inflammatory
reaction in the wall of the bowel with formation of characteristic
granulomata. Eggs may be passed in the faeces or carried to the liver
where they give rise to cirrhosis and portal hypertension with splenomegaly and ascites.

Clinical features
- Swimmer's itch: an itchy papular rash appearing 5–15 hours after
initial invasion by cercariae in previously sensitized individual.
- Katayama fever may develop 20–60 days after invasion, when
egg-laying commences, especially with S. japonicum. Fever, headache, diarrhoea, urticaria, eosinophilia, hepatosplenomegaly and
generalized lymphadenopathy. May persist for several weeks.
- Dysenteric syndrome associated with bloody diarrhoea, weight
loss, abdominal pain and moderate anaemia.
- Hepatosplenomegaly syndrome associated with less diarrhoea;
upper abdominal discomfort a major feature; progressive enlargement of liver and later spleen. Ultimately cirrhosis and portal hypertension.
- Stools contain blood, pus and mucus. Eggs present.
- Sigmoidoscopy: inflamed mucosa with haemorrhages; character-
istic eggs present in biopsy 'snips'. Later fibrosis with polyp formation.
- Marked eosinophilia.
- Occasional deposition of eggs at other sites; lungs and brain in
S. japonicum infection; spinal cord in S. mansoni infection.

Laboratory diagnosis
- Demonstration of characteristic eggs in stool; if necessary after concentration by sedimentation or centrifugation.
- Histology revealing ova in rectal 'snip'.
- Serology using Elisa (enzyme-linked immunoadsorbent assay) test is positive in more than 90% of cases and has high degree of specificity.
- High eosinophil count in peripheral blood.

Treatment
Praziquantel is effective against all human schistosomes.
- *S. mansoni*: a single oral dose of 40 mg/kg.
- *S. japonicum*: 60 mg/kg over 1 day in three divided doses by mouth.

Prevention

Immediate
- Isolation unnecessary once diagnosis has been established. Ensure hygienic disposal of faeces.
- Early treatment.
- Report to health authority.
- Contacts: search for cases and symptomless infections so that treatment can be given and possible common source identified.

Longterm
- Hygienic disposal of sewage.
- Purification of water supplies.
- Reduction of snail infestation of water courses.
- Prevention of skin exposure to contaminated water.
- Treatment of cases and carriers to prevent water contamination.

Encephalitis

The term encephalitis encompasses a wide range of pathological processes and clinical syndromes involving the brain. In many cases inflammation of the brain is accompanied by inflammation of the meninges and to a lesser extent of the spinal cord. The reaction may be generalized or focal with a varying degree of constitutional upset or involvement of other organs.

Organism/disease	Pathogenesis
Acute viral encephalitis	
Adenovirus	Transmission of virus by bloodstream
Arboviruses	or along axons. Destructive lesions in
Coxsackie virus	grey matter; patchy demyelination;
Cytomegalovirus	perivascular cuffing with mononuclear
EB (Epstein–Barr) virus	cells. Inclusion bodies in rabies and in
ECHOvirus	cytomegalovirus infections
Herpes simplex virus	
HIV	
Influenza virus A and B	
Lymphocytic choriomeningitis virus	
Mumps virus	
Poliovirus	
Rabies virus	
Post-infectious encephalitis	
Many virus infections including:	Immunological reaction in persons
Influenza	sensitized to myelin due to presence of
Measles	virus or virus antigen in tissues.
Mumps	Perivascular cuffing, microglial
Rubella	proliferation, demyelination
Varicella/zoster	characteristically perivenous
Slow-virus infections	
Measles	*Subacute sclerosing panencephalitis*:
Papovavirus	perivenous cuffing, proliferation of
Rubella	microglia and hypertrophy of
	astrocytes; little demyelination;
	inclusions present and measles virus
	recoverable on biopsy; high levels of
	measles antibody in CSF and blood.
	Similar syndrome in congenital rubella

Encephalitis

Organism/disease/pathogenesis

Organism/disease	Pathogenesis
	Progressive multifocal leucoencephalopathy: this may complicate lymphoma: focal demyelination; virus in oligodendrocytes
Viroids	
Jakob–Creutzfeldt	Brain spongy, no inflammatory
Kuru	response
Other infections	Pathology varies with infecting agent
Rickettsiae	Typhus associated with cerebral vasculitis
Tuberculosis	Tuberculosis, syphilis and fungal
Syphilis	infections accompanied by chronic
Histoplasmosis	meningitis resulting in hydrocephalus,
Cryptococcosis	gliosis and vascular damage. Thick mucoid exudate in cryptococcal infection
Mycoplasma	
Pyogenic bacteria	
Leptospirosis	
Lyme disease	
Malaria	
Toxoplasmosis	
Trypanosomiasis	
Naegleria	

Epidemiology

• Varies with different causative agents.

• Arboviruses. Mosquito-borne: equine encephalitis in North America, Japanese B encephalitis in Asia. Tick-borne: mainly Central Europe and Russia. Person-to-person transmission not described. Laboratory infections may occur.

• HIV may cause primary encephalitis (p. 137).

• Jakob–Creutzfeldt encephalitis: usually middle or old age; transmitted by direct inoculation, e.g. brain biopsy needles, injected human pituitary extract.

Encephalitis

Epidemiology

- Kuru: associated with cannibalism.
- Toxoplasmal and cryptococcal encephalitis: may occur in patients with Aids (p. 137).
- Primary amoebic meningoencephalitis: rare, mainly in young adults; associated with diving or energetic swimming in polluted warm waters.

Clinical features

Acute viral
- Brief prodromal period of fever, malaise and lassitude.
- Onset sudden or gradual.
- Illness very variable: transient drowsiness to profound coma and death.
- CNS: usually neck stiffness and drowsiness. May be no focal signs. Sometimes convulsions, ocular palsies, ataxia, hemiplegia, hypothalamic disturbance, behavioural disorders.
- CSF: usually under slightly increased pressure. Moderate number of cells, mainly mononuclear. Protein and sugar levels usually normal but may be slightly increased. Virus may be grown on culture.

Acute post-infectious
Onset 2–12 days after commencement of illness. Course very variable and similar to acute viral.

Slow-virus infections
- *Subacute sclerosing panencephalitis (SSPE)*: very rare disease of children and young adults characterized by progressive dementia, myoclonic movements and a variety of neurological signs. Usually fatal within 2 years (p. 170).
- *Jakob–Creutzfeldt disease*: progressive dementia with ataxia and myoclonus; distinctive EEG (electroencephalograph); CSF usually normal. Usually fatal within year.

Other infections
Clinical presentation and course of illness vary with the causative agent.

Treatment

Viral encephalitis
- Mainly symptomatic.
- Acyclovir should be considered for herpes simplex encephalitis.
- Corticosteroid therapy may reduce cerebral oedema but is otherwise of doubtful value.
- Zidovudine should be considered for HIV infection.

Other infections
Specific treatment should be given when indicated.

Prevention

Immediate
- Isolation: strict until causation is known, then according to disease.
- Inform health authority. Acute encephalitis notifiable in UK.
- Contacts action and other measures: see under each disease.

Longterm
- That of causative condition.
- Control of arthropod vectors.
- Growth hormone of human pituitary origin should not be prescribed.
- Primary amoebic meningoencephalitis: hygienic maintenance of swimming pools; avoid swimming in natural warm springs.
- Immunization: see under each disease and in appendix on immunization (p. 352).

Endocarditis (infective)

Clinical features

Initial illness

Onset usually gradual but may be abrupt with virulent organism. Early symptoms non-specific and resemble influenza. Arthritis and myalgia common and may be presenting symptoms. Remittent or intermittent fever with bouts of sweating or rigors. Alternating periods of fever and normal temperature in subacute variety. Fever may be absent in 5% of patients. Septicaemic illness may overshadow heart damage.

Cardiac signs

Heart murmur present in great majority of patients. Changing or new murmur highly significant but only found in small proportion. Ruptured aortic cusp may lead to rapid left ventricular failure. Congestive heart failure may develop late, even after successful antibiotic treatment.

Immune complexes

Deposition of immune complexes may give rise to petechial haemorrhages in the conjunctivae, buccal mucosa and skin, or to splinter haemorrhages under the nails. Osler's nodes, small tender nodules, may be found in the pulps of the fingers and toes. Glomerulonephritis is common.

Embolism

Major embolism occurs in 40% of patients and commonly involves kidney, spleen, brain or eye.

Other features

Continued illness may be accompanied by loss of weight and progressive anaemia. Splenomegaly and clubbing may develop in about 50% of patients.

Organism/epidemiology/pathogenesis/laboratory diagnosis

Organism/epidemiology	Pathogenesis	Laboratory diagnosis
Young adults (apart from drug addicts) • Viridans streptococci (*Strep. mutans, sanguis, milleri, mitis, bovis*) • Faecal streptococci • Others (including *Staph. epidermidis*)	Bacteraemia, with or without recognized preceding incident, in patients with predisposing heart lesions, e.g. rheumatic carditis, congenital abnormality, except atrial septal defect. Leads to deposition of organisms at site of impact; inflammatory response results in vegetation formation. *Staph. epidermidis* commonly affects bicuspid aortic valve	• Blood cultures (at least three sets, taken before starting treatment) • Microscopic haematuria (may be a late finding) • Reduced C_3 component of complement (may be a late finding) • WBC count normal or neutropenia in subacute infections; polymorphonuclear leucocytosis in acute infections • Normochromic, normocytic anaemia. Raised ESR • Infections with coxiella and chlamydia diagnosed serologically
Drug addicts • *Staph. aureus* • Faecal streptococci • Group B streptococci • *E. coli* • *Proteus* spp. • *Serratia* spp. • *Ps. aeruginosa* • Anaerobes	Predilection for tricuspid valve infection. Approx. 70% have no evidence of underlying heart disease	

Endocarditis (infective)

Organism/epidemiology/pathogenesis/laboratory diagnosis

Septicaemia with any virulent pyogenic organism can cause endocarditis in a normal heart

Adults after middle age
- Viridans streptococci
- Faecal streptococci
- Enterobacteria
- *Staph. epidermidis*

Post-cardiac surgery (early)
- *Staph. aureus*
- *Staph. epidermidis*
- Diphtheroids

Post-cardiac surgery (late)
As early and other adults, in addition
Candida spp., *Aspergillus* spp.

Culture negative
- Previous antibiotics
- *Coxiella burnetii*
- *C. psittaci*
- Fastidious streptococci
- Anaerobes

Treatment
- Initiate treatment as soon as blood cultures have been taken.
- Select antibiotic according to likely sensitivity of most probable pathogen. Modify later in light of sensitivity tests on organism cultured.
- Monitor effectiveness by determining serum concentration of antibiotic and by titrating serum against the organism. Dosage of antibiotic should be adjusted to produce bactericidal effect when serum is diluted 1 : 8.
- Bactericidal antibiotics should be used and given i.v. for 4−6 weeks according to response: benzylpenicillin for sensitive streptococci and staphylococci; flucloxacillin for resistant staphylococci; a combination of gentamicin, carbenicillin or amoxycillin for Gram-negative organisms; amphotericin B or flucytosine plus amphotericin for fungal infections; prolonged course of tetracycline for coxiella and chlamydial infections; culture-negative cases should be given combined treatment with ampicillin and gentamicin, adding metronidazole or clindamycin if an anaerobic infection seems likely (e.g. in drug addicts).
- Excise valve and replace with prosthesis in coxiella endocarditis or when valve has been grossly damaged.

Prevention
- Isolation unnecessary.
- That of primary infection.
- Chemoprophylaxis (p. 343).
- Education and therapy in i.v. drug abuse.

Enterovirus infections

Organisms

Enteroviruses (a subgroup of picornaviruses) include Coxsackie A (24 serotypes), Coxsackie B (six serotypes), ECHOvirus (34 serotypes) and polioviruses (three serotypes). Apart from Coxsackie A viruses, isolated in suckling mice, enteroviruses grow well in monkey kidney or human amnion cell lines.

Epidemiology

Distribution

Worldwide, common infections, especially in young children, who are usually symptomless. Adult infection, though less common, causes illness more frequently but is rare in areas with poor standards of hygiene and sanitation, where infection is endemic. Improvements in environmental sanitation tend to reduce endemic infection in infants and young children. However, these improvements may be followed by outbreaks of infection, with associated illness, in non-immune older children and adults who escaped infection at an earlier age. Infections most common in late summer and autumn in temperate climates; in tropical zones high incidence continues throughout the year.

Poliovirus infection: rare in communities with effective childhood immunization programmes, but may still spread within these communities causing paralytic poliomyelitis in unimmunized persons; remains common in areas of poor hygiene. In UK, average about five cases paralytic poliomyelitis per year 1970–87, about 60% due to wild virus, most in unimmunized persons, nearly 33% of which acquired overseas, about 40% associated with oral poliovirus vaccine (OPV).

Coxsackie and ECHOvirus infections: often occur in epidemics, sometimes pandemics. Usually cause benign self-limiting disease but sometimes severe, generalized infections with deaths, especially in neonates in hospital units. Chronic Coxsackie B virus infection is believed to be associated with post-viral fatigue syndrome. Virus types vary from year to year, some may be mutually exclusive; poliovirus and Coxsackie B virus infections rarely occur in the same community at the same time. High prevalence of Coxsackie or ECHOvirus infections may reduce efficiency of OPV by preventing colonization of gut by vaccine virus. Acute haemorrhagic conjunctivitis is caused by enterovirus 70 (p. 48).

Source
Human cases or inapparent infection. Virus present in throat and faeces within a few days of infection and up to 7 days before onset of symptoms; may persist in faeces for as long as 2–3 months; virus present in vesicular fluid in hand, foot and mouth disease, and in eye discharges in acute haemorrhagic conjunctivitis.

Spread
Close contact with faeces or pharyngeal secretions of infected persons, with vesicle fluid in hand, foot and mouth disease, and direct or indirect contact with eye discharges in acute haemorrhagic conjunctivitis. Usual spread by faecal–oral route.

Pathogenesis
Entry to the body is via the mouth, replication takes place in the lymphoid tissue of the gastrointestinal tract and virus is excreted in the faeces. Viraemia may occur, leading to neurological or other systemic manifestations.

Clinical features

Syndrome	Coxsackie	ECHOvirus	Poliovirus
Aseptic meningitis	A1, 2, 4, 5, 6, 7, 9, 10, 16, 22, 24 and B1–5	1–7, 9, 11–15, 17–23, 25, 30 and 31	1, 2 and 3
Paralytic disease	A4, 7, 9 and B1–5	1, 2, 4, 6, 9 and 11	1, 2 and 3
Encephalitis	A2, 5, 6, 9, B1, 2, 3 and 5	3, 4, 6, 7, 9, 11, 16, 18 and 30	1, 2 and 3
Exanthematous disease:			
• Maculopapular rashes	B5	9, 11 and 16	
• Petechial rashes	A9 and B3	4 and 9	
• Hand, foot and mouth disease	A5, 10 and 16		

Enterovirus infections

Clinical features

Syndrome	Coxsackie	ECHOvirus	Poliovirus
Upper respiratory disease:			
• Herpangina	A (all types)		
• Ulcerative stomatitis	A5 and 16		
• Lymphonodular pharyngitis	A10		
Lower respiratory disease:			
• Acute catarrh	A21 and B (all)		
• Croup		11	
• Pneumonitis, pleurisy	A9 and B (all)	9	
Epidemic myalgia (Bornholm)	B (all types)		
Pericarditis and myocarditis	B1−5		
Generalized disease in the newborn	B (all types), A (some suspected)	11 and possibly others	
Respiratory-enteric disease		8, 11, 19 and 20	
Gastroenteritis		11, 14 and 18	
Hepatitis:			
• Neonates	B (all types)		
• Older children	A and B		
Ocular disease			
• Conjunctivitis	A9, 16 and B5	1, 4, 6, 9, 16 and 20	
• Nodular conjunctivitis	A10		
Orchitis	B5		
Lymphadenitis and splenomegaly	A5, 6 and B5		

Bornholm disease
- Incubation period 2−5 days.
- Disabling pain on one side of lower chest or upper abdomen, griping, continuous or spasmodic, aggravated by deep breathing or

movement. Myalgia of trunk, neck and limbs not infrequent. Duration 2−3 weeks.
- Fever during spasms. Malaise and headaches, few other symptoms.
- Myocarditis, encephalitis and orchitis present in some.

Hand, foot and mouth disease
- Incubation period 3−7 days.
- Children more frequently affected than adults.
- Fever and slight malaise.
- Sore mouth. Bright red macules, small vesicles or shallow painful ulcers present in all parts of the mouth but seldom on tonsils and not on pharynx.
- Rash consists of erythematous macules, small vesicles, thin bullae or grey ulcers within erythematous base. Rash on hands mainly on sides of fingers; rash on feet found particularly on toes and lateral aspect, but seldom present in children under the age of 3; maculopapular rash may be present on buttocks of young children.

Herpangina
- Incubation period 2−10 days.
- Onset abrupt with sore throat, fever and vomiting.
- Throat reddened and discrete lesions present on anterior pillar of fauces, palate and uvula; greyish papules surrounded by erythematous zone, also shallow ulcers up to 5 mm across, usually between five and ten lesions.
- Duration of illness about 4 days.

Poliomyelitis
- Incubation period varies from 3−35 days, average 10−15 days.
- Abortive or minor attack presents as influenzal illness or as tonsilitis with generalized lymphadenopathy or as gastroenteritis. Fever subsides after 4−5 days or longer.
- Aseptic meningitis is a more severe form terminating without paralysis.
- Paralytic disease may be spinal, bulbospinal or encephalitic according to part of nervous system chiefly affected. Initial presentation is that of aseptic meningitis followed by secondary rise of temperature with the onset of flaccid paralysis. Paralysis is maximal at the

end of febrile phase. Thereafter, some degree of recovery may be expected over a period of 1 year to 18 months. Paralysis of swallowing or breathing may endanger life. Paralysis of the bladder recovers within a week or two.

Laboratory diagnosis
• Asymptomatic gastrointestinal infection is common. Virus isolation from throat washings or faeces should be supported by demonstration of a rising titre of neutralizing humoral antibody for confirmation of systemic infection.
• Virus isolation from CSF should be attempted in aseptic meningitis and encephalitis, but CSF cultures are not positive in paralytic poliomyelitis.
• Serodiagnosis is impracticable because of the multiplicity of enterovirus serotypes.

Treatment — poliomyelitis
• Bedrest and analgesics.
• Postural drainage and tube-feeding for pharyngeal paralysis.
• Ventilation for respiratory paralysis.
• Intermittent catherization for bladder paralysis.
• Active physiotherapy for residual weakness in skeletal muscles.

Prevention

Immediate — poliomyelitis
• Isolation: enteric precautions in hospital until stools negative for poliovirus. If virus culture not available isolate arbitrarily for 3 weeks.
• Inform health authority; notifiable in UK. Paralytic cases should be reported to World Health Organization (WHO).
• Search for possible source by identifying missed cases.
• Contacts among household and health-care staff: faeces or rectal swab and throat swab to identify virus causing index case, then OPV to block spread of virus (ring immunization), exclusion from work or school until after OPV.
• Mass immunization. Consider OPV for school or work contacts. Community immunization should be considered if two or more paralytic cases in a locality.

Prevention

Immediate — enterovirus infection in neonatal unit
- Isolation: enteric precautions of cases and ward contacts.
- Inform hospital control-of-infection officer.
- Scrupulous hygiene to prevent faecal–oral spread.
- Close unit to new admissions if second case occurs.
- Contacts: immunization with OPV should be considered as a means of possibly blocking spread of virus, especially Coxsackie B.

Immediate — other enterovirus infections
- Isolation: in hospital, enteric and wound precautions.
- Hand, foot and mouth disease: exclude cases from school or work whilst skin lesions are present.

Longterm
- Good hygiene. Avoidance of contact with pharyngeal secretions.
- Routine immunization against poliomyelitis in childhood with reinforcing doses when visiting endemic areas (p. 357).

Food poisoning

1 Botulism

Organism

Clostridium botulinum: anaerobic, Gram-positive spore-bearing rod: distinct strains distinguished by the antigenic type of the potent neurotoxin produced; types A, B and E of importance to man.

Epidemiology

Distribution
Worldwide, rare disease caused by the ingestion of preformed toxin from *Cl. botulinum* types A, B and E; sporadic cases and small outbreaks occur; affects mainly adults; high mortality. In UK 26 cases with 15 deaths in nine separate episodes, 1925–87; more frequent in North America, continental Europe and Japan. Infection with *Cl. botulinum* and subsequent absorption of toxin may occur; wound botulism in adults very rare (see sporing anaerobes, p. 5); infant botulism after ingestion of organisms, about 70 cases per year in USA 1980–85, only two reported in UK.

Source
Cl. botulinum types A and B widespread in environment; type E in fish.

Spread
Raw or undercooked contaminated foods; contamination after cooking; storage under anaerobic conditions with inadequate refrigeration. Commonly home-canned vegetables in USA, smoked or cured meats in northern Europe, vegetables in southern Europe, fish in Japan. Unusual vehicles in recently reported common-source outbreaks in North America; sauté onions, garlic in soyabean oil, baked potatoes, meat pies, beef stew and turkey loaf. Infant botulism in USA has been associated with consumption of honey. Not communicable from person to person.

Pathogenesis
Spores of *Cl. botulinum* convert to vegetative (bacillary) form in food under anaerobic conditions, multiply and produce exotoxin, which is

ingested and absorbed. The toxin acts by blocking acetylcholine released at synapses and neuromuscular junctions, resulting in paralysis.

Clinical features
- Incubation is usually 5–36 hours but may extend from 5 hours to 8 days.

Older children and adults
- Severity very variable.
- Nausea, vomiting. No diarrhoea. Eventual ileus.
- Weakness, dizziness, dry mouth, postural hypotension.
- Afebrile.
- Progressive paralysis: ocular, bulbar, limb, respiratory. No sensory loss.
- Death may result from respiratory failure or inhalation pneumonia.
- Recovery very gradual.

Infants
- Constipation followed 3–10 days later by feeding difficulty.
- Irritability.
- Hoarse cry. Weakness. Cranial nerve palsies. Respiratory failure.
- Most recover spontaneously.

Laboratory diagnosis
Exotoxin demonstrable in patient's serum and occasionally in vomitus by protection studies in mice; also demonstrable in residual food if available.

Treatment
- Trivalent antitoxin A, B and E. Equine more readily available than human. Half the dose should be given i.v. and half i.m.
- Supportive measures may include tracheostomy, artificial ventilation and nasogastric or i.v. feeding.

Prevention
See below, p. 92.

2 Staphylococcal

Organism
Staphylococcus aureus: enterotoxin-producing strains (p. 271).

Epidemiology

Distribution
Worldwide, common; usually outbreaks, sporadic cases rarely detected; caused by ingestion of preformed enterotoxin. Incidence highest in warm weather; declining in UK, less than 20 outbreaks reported annually 1980–87.

Source
Staphylococcal skin lesions of infected food handler, less commonly nasal carrier. Rarely mastitis in cattle.

Spread
Manual contamination by infected food handler; often cooked or preserved salted meats, such as ham, subsequently stored at room temperature for at least 6 hours, or inadequately refrigerated. Raw milk and dairy products. Not communicable from person to person.

Pathogenesis
Exotoxin produced by contaminating staphylococci diffuses into foodstuff and is ingested. The toxin is absorbed and stimulates first the neuroreceptors in the gut and then the gut motility centres in the medulla. Vomiting, often projectile, is induced.

Clinical features
- Incubation period: 1–6 hours.
- Abrupt onset.
- Severe vomiting followed by variable diarrhoea.
- Recovery in 6–24 hours.

Laboratory diagnosis
- Heating food before consumption may kill *Staph. aureus* without destruction of exotoxin.

Laboratory diagnosis

• Recovery of organism from vomitus or faeces should be attempted but may not be successful.

• Any strain of *Staph. aureus* from food or clinical specimens should be examined for exotoxin production; testing usually carried out in specialist laboratories. Phage typing important for epidemiological investigation of source and spread of the disease.

Treatment
• Maintain water and electrolyte balance.
• Metoclopramide.
• Diphenoxylate or loperamide.

Prevention
See below, p. 92.

3 *Bacillus cereus*

Organism
Bacillus cereus: aerobic, Gram-positive, spore-bearer, enterotoxin-producing strains.

Epidemiology

Distribution
Worldwide with large geographic variations. Usually toxin (short incubation) type disease in UK with up to 30 outbreaks reported annually 1980−87; both toxin and infection (long incubation) types common in continental Europe; rare in USA. Wound infection with *B. cereus* has been described and may be common in the tropics.

Source
Soil and environment. Widespread in cereals and cereal products.

Spread
Foods: commonly rice dishes, moistened and kept without refriger-ation under warm conditions for several hours. Not transmissible from person to person.

Pathogenesis
Ingestion of preformed enterotoxin (short incubation period), or of organisms which produce enterotoxin during growth in the gut (longer incubation period).

Clinical features

Toxin
- Incubation period: 1−6 hours.
- Vomiting, abdominal pain and slight diarrhoea.

Infection
- Incubation period: 8−16 hours.
- Abdominal pain and diarrhoea lasting 12−24 hours.

Laboratory diagnosis
Organism recoverable from infected foodstuffs and usually from excreta; tests for toxin production carried out in specialist laboratories.

Treatment
See staphylococcal food poisoning, p. 86.

Prevention
See below, p. 92.

4 *Clostridium perfringens*

Organism
Clostridium perfringens: enterotoxin-producing strains, the majority producing heat-resistant spores.

Epidemiology

Distribution
Worldwide; varies with practices in food preparation; in UK 50−80 outbreaks reported every year 1980−87, mostly in institutions. A very

rare severe necrotizing enterocolitis has been described in mal-nourished populations ('pigbel' in New Guinea).

Source
Gastrointestinal tract of animals; raw meats.

Spread
Usually reheated meat dishes, contaminated before or after cooking and stored without refrigeration at room temperature and slowly reheated. Not transmissible from person to person.

Pathogenesis
Ingestion of vegetative organisms in contaminated food; sporulation, with elaboration and release of enterotoxin, follows; enterotoxin causes hypersecretion in jejunum and ileum and thus diarrhoea.

Clinical features
- Incubation period: 12–20 hours.
- Abdominal colic.
- Moderate diarrhoea but seldom vomiting.
- Duration about 3 days.

Laboratory diagnosis
- Semiqualitative methods applied to differentiate between faecal commensals and food poisoning (in food poisoning usually $>10^6$ *Cl. perfringens*/g faeces).
- Cultures should include methods for recognition of both heat-resistant spores (i.e. survive 100°C for 60 minutes) and more heat-sensitive strains.
- In outbreaks, isolation of same serotype is expected from majority of specimens.

Treatment
Symptomatic.

Prevention
See below, p. 92.

5 Salmonella
See p. 246.

6 *Vibrio parahaemolyticus*

Organism
Vibrio parahaemolyticus: curved, Gram-negative, aerobic rod, differentiated from *V. cholerae* by biochemical and serological reactions.

Epidemiology

Distribution
Common in warm climates in populations consuming seafoods, especially Japan, South East Asia and parts of USA; highest incidence in summer. Rare in UK, up to 20 cases reported annually 1980−87, mostly infected abroad.

Source
Fish, shellfish and marine environment.

Spread
Raw seafood, cross-contamination of cooked foods from contaminated raw fish, shellfish or seawater, and subsequent inadequate refrigeration or storage at room temperature. Not communicable from person to person.

Pathogenesis
Organisms invade superficial mucosal cells in small intestine: precise aetiology of resulting diarrhoea not understood.

Clinical features
- Incubation period: 10−20 hours.
- Abrupt onset.
- Vomiting, diarrhoea and abdominal pain.
- Recovery: few days.

Laboratory diagnosis
Isolate on same selective media as *V. cholerae*; differentiation by fermentation reactions.

Prevention
See below, p. 99.

7 Viral

Organisms
Over 90% of cases associated with small round viruses, including parvoviruses, and also calicivirus.

Epidemiology

Distribution
Probably worldwide; incidence apparently increasing in UK, around 20 outbreaks reported annually 1980–87, often associated with consumption of undercooked or raw shellfish and raw vegetables.

Source
Human.

Spread
Sewage pollution of shellfish beds and of irrigation water causing contamination of shellfish and vegetables. Direct contamination of food from faecally contaminated hands of infected food handlers.

Pathogenesis
Following ingestion, viruses replicate in small-intestinal epithelial cells. Resulting damage reduces absorptive capacity of gut and causes diarrhoea. Pathogenesis of associated vomiting not understood.

Clinical features
- Incubation period: about 36 hours.
- Rapid onset.
- Vomiting in 50%; diarrhoea 75%; abdominal cramps.

Clinical features

- Fever minimal; some have flu-like illness.
- Duration: 1–2 days with rapid recovery.

Laboratory diagnosis
Demonstration of virus particles in faeces by electron microscopy; specimens should be obtained early in the disease.

Treatment
Symptomatic.

Prevention
See below, p. 99.

8 Toxic substances

Epidemiology/clinical features

Distribution
Worldwide; varies with food habits. Rapid onset of symptoms within minutes or 1–2 hours of consumption of toxic substance; usually quick recovery. Most types of toxic food poisoning are rare.

Type	Epidemiology	Clinical features
Fish	• Scombroid poisoning due to histamine-like substances in spoiled scombroid fish (mackerel, tuna), but other types of fish may be involved. Increase in UK in 1980s, up to 20 episodes reported a year	Hot flushing, headache, diarrhoea. Recovery in few hours
	• Ciguatera poisoning due to various fish of coral reefs. Mainly Caribbean	Paraesthesia, numbness, vomiting, diarrhoea. Recovery may take several weeks
	• Tetraodon poisoning due to toxic puffer fish. Mainly Japan	Numbness, weakness, vomiting, diarrhoea, paralysis, coma. High mortality

Food poisoning: Toxic substances

Epidemiology/clinical features

Type	Epidemiology	Clinical features
Shellfish	• Paralytic shellfish poisoning due to mussels, which have fed on toxin-producing dinoflagellates of genus *Gonyaulax*. Occurs in temperate zones • Red whelk poisoning, salivary glands of red whelk, *Neptuna antigua*, produce toxin tetramine	Paraesthesia, numbness, headache, weakness, paresis. Recovery usual but may be fatal Nausea, vomiting, blurred vision, weakness and paralysis. Recovery within 1–2 days usual
Metallic	Usually due to preparation or storage of acid foods in zinc- or copper-lined containers	Sudden vomiting. Recovery usual within a few hours
Mushroom	Due to poisonous fungi of species *Amanita*, containing muscarine or amantadine	Abdominal pain, vomiting, diarrhoea, convulsions, coma. High mortality
Potato	Solanine in skin of sprouting potatoes, or tubers exposed to light during growth	Headache, vomiting, diarrhoea, weakness. Recovery usual within 3–4 days
Red bean	Heat-labile toxin present in raw or undercooked kidney beans	Nausea, vomiting, diarrhoea. Recovery within a few hours

Prevention

Outbreaks should be investigated in conjunction with a microbiologist and environmental health physician to ensure that appropriate specimens are examined: foodstuffs likely to be responsible, faeces and sometimes vomitus are tested. Ideally samples of food prepared in hospitals, institutions and catering should be refrigerated and kept for at least 48 hours to facilitate investigation of any related outbreak of food poisoning. Aerobic and anaerobic cultures of foodstuffs are incubated on appropriate media; quantitative methods are usually employed.

Food poisoning: Toxic substances

Prevention

Immediate
- Isolation: enteric precautions until diagnosis established. Continue isolation for salmonella and viral food poisoning; unnecessary for other causes.
- Report to health authority (by telephone in suspected botulism); notifiable in UK.
- Identify persons possibly exposed to same source of infection for epidemiological investigation. In botulism, contacts known to have consumed contaminated food should have gastric lavage, purgation and high enemas, and should be kept under close medical observation; antitoxin should be given immediately if symptoms develop. Antitoxin should also be used for prophylaxis if it is considered that the risk of botulism is high.
- Obtain samples of suspected food vehicles for examination. In salmonella food poisoning, environmental swabs of tables, slicing machines, refrigerators and drain swabs usually valuable.
- Clinical examination of catering staff in staphylococcal food poisoning to find infected skin lesions and collect swabs of lesions and nose for culture. Exclude from work until healed. Faecal specimens from kitchen staff in salmonella food poisoning to confirm association with catering premises; excreters are more likely to be the result rather than the cause of outbreak.
- Cases and excreters of salmonellae; exclude from work food handlers and health-care staff in whom there may be high risk of spread, until three bacteriologically negative faeces specimens collected at intervals of not less than 24 hours (see salmonellosis, p. 249).

Longterm
- Continuing education of the public and employees in the food industry in personal and food hygiene.
- Separation of cooked foods from raw materials.
- Adequate cooking before eating.
- Rapid cooling of cooked foods and refrigeration at about +4°C until required for eating.
- Full thawing of frozen foods before cooking.
- Frequent inspection of hygiene of catering staff and kitchen premises to identify and rectify faults.
- Pasteurization of milk, dairy products and bulk egg products.
- Control of salmonellosis in animals (p. 250).

Gastroenteritis

General

Gastroenteritis varies greatly according to the aetiology of the infection and the age of the patient. In infants and young children, vomiting and diarrhoea rapidly lead to dehydration and imbalance of electrolytes, consequently gastroenteritis is a serious disease with an appreciable mortality. In older children and adults the illness may be incapacitating but is seldom fatal. The clinical features of many types of gastroenteritis are very similar and it is difficult on clinical evaluation to be certain of the nature of the infection. Laboratory investigation is essential to establish the cause so that appropriate measures can be taken to trace the source of infection and prevent further spread. Maintenance of fluid balance is the most important aspect of treatment and antibiotic therapy is seldom beneficial.

1 Campylobacter

Organism

Campylobacters: vibrio-like, microaerophilic, Gram-negative organisms; optimal growth at 42°C. Two species, *C. jejuni* and *C. coli*, can cause infection of the small intestine; another campylobacter-like organism, *C. pyloridis*, described in early 1980s in association with gastritis.

Epidemiology

Distribution

Worldwide, very common; affects all age groups; mostly sporadic, but common-source outbreaks frequently reported. First recognized as a cause of acute diarrhoeal disease in man in early 1970s; now the most frequently isolated pathogen in many countries, nearly 25 000 reports in UK in 1987. Probably an important cause of traveller's diarrhoea.

The aetiological role and epidemiology of *C. pyloridis* in gastritis, gastric and duodenal ulceration not yet clear.

Gastroenteritis: Campylobacter

Epidemiology

Source
Farm livestock, particularly poultry; possibly environmental in water.
Viable organisms may be non-culturable.

Spread
Foodborne, often associated with fresh untrussed poultry; milkborne
outbreaks due to unpasteurized milk common; waterborne outbreaks
have been described. Direct contact with infected animals, especially
puppies and kittens. Person-to-person spread appears rare. Contamination of food from food handlers, who are excreters of the organism, has not been described.

Pathogenesis
Characteristically cause jejunoileitis with mucosal oedema and
polymorphonuclear infiltration; sometimes microabscesses; procto-
colitis may occur. Pathogenesis is not known.

Clinical features
- Incubation period; usually 5 days, may extend from 2 to 11 days.
- Low-grade fever and malaise for 2–3 days before diarrhoea.
- Headache, myalgia, nausea, vomiting, occasional rigor.
- Profuse diarrhoea lasting 1–3 days; sometimes blood and mucus
in stool.
- Severe abdominal pain may mimic appendicitis.
- Septicaemia and arthritis in about 1–2% of cases.
- Continuing malaise and colic over a period of 10–14 days.

Laboratory diagnosis
Isolation of organism from faeces on antibiotic-containing selective
medium, incubated under reduced oxygen tension at 42°C; identification by colonial and microscopic morphology and by inability of
subculture to grow in air.

Treatment
- Symptomatic for mild attack.
- Erythromycin 1 g daily in severe attack; also tetracycline or
neomycin.
- Gentamicin effective alternative for septicaemia.

Prevention

Immediate
- Isolation: enteric precautions in hospital whilst symptoms persist.
- Report clusters of cases to health authority for epidemiological investigation. In UK notifiable only if believed to be foodborne, as 'food poisoning'.
- Contacts: bacteriological screening unnecessary except for epidemiological purposes.
- Exclusion of recovered cases and symptomless excreters from food handling or other work is not justified.

Longterm
- Hygienic production of poultry.
- Food hygiene to prevent cross-contamination to other foods, particularly cooked foods and salads.
- Pasteurization of milk and dairy products.
- Purification and disinfection of water supplies.
- Care in handling sick pets and other animals.

2 *Escherichia coli*

Organisms
Escherichia coli: strains with ability to cause gastroenteritis fall into three groups: enteropathogenic (EPEC), enterotoxic (ETEC) and enteroinvasive (EIEC). EPEC recognized by serological identification of O antigens; relatively few O types cause disease. Recognition of ETEC and EIEC strains by demonstrating toxin production or invasion of mucosa following injection into isolated segments of rabbit intestine, or for ETEC strains, cytotoxic effect in tissue culture. In addition verotoxin-producing strains (VTEC) have been associated with haemorrhagic colitis (p. 38) and with haemolytic uraemic syndrome (p. 110).

Epidemiology

Distribution
Worldwide. EPEC strains cause infantile gastroenteritis, common in areas of poor hygiene. ETEC strains cause traveller's diarrhoea, all ages. EIEC cause dysentery-like syndrome in older children and adults. VTEC strains reported in UK, North America and Japan.

Source
Human cases and excreters.

Spread
EPEC and EIEC: usually person-to-person spread by faecal−oral route; outbreaks in hospitals and nurseries common. ETEC: usually foodborne or waterborne, outbreaks associated with milk and cheese have been reported. VTEC: foodborne, particularly meat products; person-to-person spread by faecal−oral route.

Pathogenesis
EPEC: enterotoxins not yet identified, but clinical features suggest this mode of action.
ETEC: heat-labile (LT) and heat-stable (ST) toxins demonstrable; either or both produced by enterotoxigenic strains, both plasmid-mediated. LT antigenically related to cholera exotoxin, and thought to act similarly (p. 35). Action of ST somewhat different; causes watery diarrhoea with little abdominal pain; no inflammatory exudate. Usually mild disease, occasionally severe and cholera-like. To cause disease ETEC strains also require fimbriae to attach to mucosal cells, and host cells must have specific receptors.

Clinical features

Infantile gastroenteritis
- Incubation: usually 2−3 days.
- Onset varies in severity; infant listless, irritable and refuses feeds.
- Vomiting and diarrhoea. Usually afebrile.
- Abdominal distension and colic.

Clinical features

- Stools watery with musty odour. Contain mucus and may be bloodstreaked.
- Dehydration and acidosis.
- Secondary infection may occur in respiratory tract and middle ears.
- Convalescence slow; may be complicated by lactose intolerance.

Other infections
Traveller's diarrhoea due to ETEC has no characteristic features. Disease associated with EIEC resembles bacillary dysentery.

Laboratory diagnosis
EPEC: faeces cultured by routine methods for intestinal pathogens; strains recognized by slide agglutination with type-specific antisera. Confirmation of slide-positive results must be obtained in a series of tube dilutions.
Other strains: not routinely identified.

Treatment
- Oral rehydration with glucose/electrolyte solution.
- Intravenous infusion may be required in severe cases.
- Graduated feeding.
- Lactose-free feeds may be required during convalescence.

Prevention

Immediate
- Isolation: enteric precautions in hospital.
- Report to hospital control-of-infection officer.
- Report clusters of cases to health authority for epidemiological investigation.
- In nurseries, and in children's and infants' wards in hospital, consider closure if two or more cases occur.

Longterm
- Meticulous hygiene in preparation of bottle feeds for infants.
- Isolation of infants/children on admission to hospital has been suggested. Probably only necessary in patients with history of diarrhoea.
- Education on hygiene to prevent faecal−oral spread.

3 Viral

Organisms
Several small viruses not yet grown in tissue culture (also implicated in winter vomiting disease) including:
- Rotavirus (wheel-like), 64 nm diameter, similar to orbivirus group of reoviruses.
- Astrovirus (five- or six-pointed star), 28 nm diameter.
- Calicivirus (calyx) 30 nm diameter with cup-like surface depressions.
- Parvovirus (small round viruses).
- Viruses commonly associated with respiratory tract infections, e.g. adenoviruses and coronaviruses.

Epidemiology

Distribution
Rotavirus: worldwide; common in infants and young children but may occur at any age; mostly sporadic but outbreaks in children's homes and hospitals common; may also occur in geriatric units; incidence highest in winter months in temperate climates; in UK over 7000 infections reported in 1987, over 90% less than 5 years of age.
Adenovirus: some types of non-culturable adenovirus, particularly types 40 and 41, cause gastroenteritis similar to rotavirus; mainly affects children under 2 years of age and has no important seasonal variation.
Norwalk agent and other small round viruses (parvovirus): cause winter vomiting disease and foodborne gastroenteritis (see viral food poisoning, p. 90).

Source
Human.

Spread
Faecal—oral route, especially in infants, young children and old people in institutions. Norwalk and other small round viruses may be foodborne, especially by shellfish harvested from sewage-polluted estuaries, or waterborne.

Pathogenesis

Rotavirus replicates within the epithelial cells of the small bowel causing destruction of the brush border with resultant deficiency of disaccharidases including lactase. Failure to digest and absorb disaccharides results in watery diarrhoea. The pathophysiology of other virus infection is poorly understood; the virus presumably replicates within intestinal mucosal cells, causing superficial damage and possibly deficient production of enzymes. Diarrhoea probably persists until the epithelium is restored. Humoral antibodies are formed, and the virus therefore presumably spreads to regional lymphatics.

Clinical features

Rotavirus
- Incubation period: 2–6 days
- Vomiting may be present for up to 48 hours before onset of diarrhoea.
- Diarrhoea very variable and may be minimal in older children. Duration may extend from 2 to 23 days.
- Fever often exceeds 38.5°C.
- General symptoms of headache and myalgia.
- Respiratory symptoms in 40% of cases; lung involvement on chest X-ray examination in 8%.
- Metabolic acidosis common.

Norwalk and related viruses
- Incubation period: 24–72 hours.
- Vomiting sometimes severe.
- Diarrhoea usually lasts for 18–36 hours.
- General symptoms of headache and myalgia.

Adenoviruses
- Incubation period: 8–10 days.
- Fever in 40–90% of cases, lasting 2–3 days.
- Diarrhoea less severe than in rotavirus infection: may last for 7–8 days; stools watery but no blood.

Clinical features

- Vomiting in 80%; occurs 1−2 days after onset of diarrhoea; usually mild and lasts for about 2 days.
- Respiratory symptoms variable.

Laboratory diagnosis
Virus particles detected by electron microscopy of faeces during acute stage. During convalescence, antibody is demonstrable by ability of serum to agglutinate faecal virus particles (immune electron microscopy).

Treatment
Symptomatic. Maintain water and electrolyte balance.

Prevention
As *E. coli* gastroenteritis, see above. See also food poisoning, p. 92.

4 Cryptosporidial

Organism
Cryptosporidium: coccidian protozoan with a complete life cycle in the gastrointestinal tract of a single host. Able to infect a wide range of animals, probably with little host specificity. Ingested oocysts undergo digestion, liberating sporozoites which enter intestinal epithelial cells and, at the cell surface, mature to form trophozoites. Trophozoites multiply asexually forming merozoites, which are discharged into the gut lumen and infect further epithelial cells. Eventually some merozoites form gametes. These fuse into zygotes and mature to oocysts, in which form they are discharged in the faeces.

Epidemiology

Distribution
Recognized as an intestinal pathogen in the late 1970s and early 1980s in immunocompromised patients, and an important manifestation of Aids; in 1983 found to be a common cause of diarrhoeal illness in immunocompetent persons. Probably worldwide distri-

bution; most frequently affects young children but occurs in all age groups. In UK over 4000 reported infections in 1987, over 40% in children less than 5 years of age.

Source
Probably mainly zoonotic, cattle and other domestic animals and pets. Occasionally human case or excreter.

Spread
Direct contact with infected animals. Waterborne outbreaks have been reported; may be milkborne or foodborne. Person-to-person spread by faecal—oral route has been described in nurseries. Spread by sexual contact in homosexuals.

Pathogenesis
Infection may extend throughout the gastrointestinal tract; cryptosporidia have also been demonstrated by lung biopsy in the immunocompromised. Infection is commonly severest in the lower jejunum and ileum, where it causes stunting and fusion of villi accompanied by local mild or moderate inflammatory cell infiltration. Mucosal dysfunction follows, with malabsorptive diarrhoea, probably due to reduction of available mucosal surface. Mixed infections with giardia or bacterial pathogens, such as campylobacter, are sometimes recorded.

Clinical features
- Incubation period: 1—10 days, usually nearer 1 than 10.
- Abdominal pain common and may precede onset of diarrhoea. May be severe and suggest possibility of appendicitis.
- Diarrhoea variable and commonly persists for 3—10 days. Stools rarely contain blood. Diarrhoea may be prolonged and severe in patients with immune deficiency.
- Sometimes associated with fever, nausea and lymphadenopathy in immunocompromised.

Laboratory diagnosis
Demonstration by microscopy of faecal oocysts, usually by staining with modified Ziehl—Nielsen or auramine methods. Direct examin-

ation of faeces is adequate during acute disease, but specimens should be concentrated to demonstrate persistence of oocysts during convalescence.

Treatment
- Specific therapy unsatisfactory and seldom necessary for self-limiting condition. May be indicated in immunocompromised patients with severe or prolonged diarrhoea.
- Spiramycin 2–4 g daily for 2–6 weeks.
- Pyrimethamine 25–50 mg, and sulphadimidine or sulphadiazine 4–8 g daily for 2–4 weeks.

Prevention

Immediate
- Isolation: enteric precautions in hospital.
- Report case clusters to health authority to enable epidemiological investigation.
- Contacts: laboratory screening not necessary except for epidemiological purposes.
- Exclusion from work or school unnecessary when symptomless.

Longterm
- Education in personal hygiene to prevent faecal–oral spread.
- Water supplies; slow filtration through fine filters to remove cysts not affected by chlorination.
- Care in handling sick animals.

Giardiasis

Organism
Giardia lamblia: protozoan found in two forms, a flagellated pear-shaped trophozoite and an ovoid cyst, the infective form.

Epidemiology

Distribution
Infection worldwide, affects all age groups with highest incidence in children; frequent cause of traveller's diarrhoea. Nearly 5000 reported infections in UK in 1987. Infection occasionally associated with dysgammaglobulinaemia.

Source
Not fully known. Animals, possibly beavers in North America. Human cases or excreters.

Spread
Waterborne outbreaks reported in North America, appear rare in UK; possibly foodborne; person-to-person spread by faecal−oral route. Homosexual activity.

Pathogenesis
Inhabits the lumen of the upper small intestine; invasion of tissue does not occur but, in heavy infections, trophozoites coat the mucosal surface of the flattened villi.

Clinical features

Symptomless
Light infection.

Acute
Incubation period about 2 weeks. Sudden onset of offensive, watery diarrhoea with much flatulence and marked abdominal distention; nausea and anorexia.

Chronic
Insidious onset or following acute episode; intermittent bouts of

Clinical features

diarrhoea with loose, yellowish greasy stools; flatulence, lassitude, weight loss; particularly common in children.

Complications
Lactose intolerance; malabsorption of fat.

Laboratory diagnosis
Demonstration of trophozoites or cysts in faeces; trophozoites usually seen only in acute infections.

Treatment
- Metronidazole 200 mg three times a day by mouth for 14 days or 2 g daily for 3 days; *or*
- Tinidazole 2 g as single dose by mouth.
- Mepacrine 100 mg three times a day by mouth for 5−8 days or chloroquine base 300 mg by mouth daily for 5 days are less effective.

Prevention

Immediate
- Isolation: enteric precautions in hospital whilst diarrhoea persists.
- Report case clusters to health authority to enable epidemiological investigation.
- Exclusion of recovered cases and cyst excreters from work or school unnecessary.

Longterm
- Purification of water supplies by filtration; cysts not affected by chlorination.
- Hygienic sewage disposal.

Gonorrhoea

Organism

Neisseria gonorrhoeae: Gram-negative diplococcus with fastidious growth requirements; human parasite which, outside the host, succumbs rapidly to dryness or cold.

Epidemiology

Distribution

Infection worldwide; commonest in young adults, rise in incidence in many countries in the 1960s and 1970s. Since 1982 homosexually acquired gonorrhoea has declined in areas affected by the Aids pandemic, following publicity about the mode of spread, with evidence of changes in sexual behaviour. However, heterosexually transmitted infection may be increasing in young people.

Penicillinase-producing *N. gonorrhoeae* first appeared in the Far East, spread to Africa, USA and Europe in the mid 1970s, continual increase in reported cases in USA but decline in UK in 1985 and 1986. Strains also resistant to spectinomycin reported. Other non-penicillinase-producing strains exhibiting high resistance to penicillin reported in USA in 1984–85.

Gonococcal ophthalmia uncommon, less frequent than chlamydial infection. Other non-sexually acquired infection rare.

Source

Human case, commonly symptomless infections in females which may persist for long periods.

Spread

Sexual contact. Ophthalmia by direct contact with infected birth canal. Rare person-to-person spread in young girls by contaminated moist objects, such as flannels and towels.

Pathogenesis

Organism attaches to columnar cells of mucous membranes, of the anterior urethra in the male, the urethra and cervix in the female, with local inflammatory response; extension via anatomical pathways causing epididymitis or salpingitis may follow, occasionally bacteraemia.

Clinical features

Incubation period
Usually 2−7 days.

Men
- *Urethritis*: scanty mucoid discharge becoming copious, purulent and sometimes bloodstained. Painful micturition. Retention of urine in severe cases. Painful lymphadenitis in 15% of cases, asymptomatic in 5%.
- *Proctitis*: homosexuals. Symptoms mild or absent. Anal dampness, pruritus or discomfort. White or yellowish discharge, sometimes bloodstained.

Women
- *Cervix and urethra*: symptoms absent in 80%. Cervix may have normal appearance with mucoid discharge or be inflamed with mucopurulent or profuse purulent discharge, sometimes bloodstained. Urethra infected from vaginal discharge; dysuria.
- *Proctitis*: rectum infected by intercourse or from vulval discharge. Symptoms as in male.
- *Local abscess*: Skene's or Bartholin's glands.
- *Pelvic spread*: endometritis, salpingitis, peritonitis.
- *Vulvovaginitis*: young girls before puberty.

Both sexes
- *Disseminated*: commoner in women than men. Bacteraemia leading to septic arthritis, tenosynovitis, endocarditis, meningitis or skin lesions.
- *Tonsillitis or pharyngitis*: especially in pregnant women.
- *Conjunctivitis*: ophthalmia neonatorum 2−5 days after birth; may give rise to septicaemia. Transfer of infection to eyes in adults.

Laboratory diagnosis

Microscopy
Demonstration of characteristic Gram-negative intracellular diplococci in urethral exudate very successful in men, less satisfactory in

women; staining with fluorescent antibody used by some workers. Infection at other sites cannot be recognized by stained smears.

Culture
Necessary in all cases for full identification and for antibiotic sensitivity testing. Specimens should be inoculated immediately onto chocolate blood agar, incorporating antibiotics to suppress the commensal flora. Incubation, in air plus 1.0% CO_2, should not be delayed. If immediate culture is impossible, then a transport medium is mandatory.

Serology
Humoral antibody detection is of no value in superficial infection and of limited usefulness in systemic infection.

Treatment

Penicillin-sensitive strains
● Procaine penicillin, single i.m. injection with probenicid 1 g orally — males 2.4 g; females 4.8 g.
● Amoxycillin or ampicillin 2 g orally with probenicid 1 g orally.
● Co-trimoxazole, two tablets twice daily or tetracycline 500 mg four times a day orally for 5 days when patient is hypersensitive to penicillin.

Penicillin-resistant strains
Spectinomycin by single i.m. injection — males 2 g; females 4 g.

Prevention

Immediate
● Isolation unnecessary for most cases; wound precautions for young children with vulvovaginitis.
● Early specific treatment.
● Report to health authority or STD clinic.
● Contacts: identification and surveillance; prophylactic treatment of contacts with or without symptoms recommended (epidemiological treatment).

Prevention

Longterm
- Health education.
- Effective early treatment.
- Prophylaxis in infants exposed to infection at birth.

Haemolytic uraemic syndrome

Organism
Diarrhoeal prodrome has been associated with a wide variety of organisms including shigella, salmonella, campylobacter, yersinia, enteroviruses and recently verotoxin-producing strains of *E. coli* (VTEC).

Epidemiology

Distribution
First described 1955, since reported in many countries; affects mainly children but adult cases occur, particularly in women during pregnancy. Usually sporadic, occasionally outbreaks. In UK about 120 cases per year reported in children; peak incidence July–August; at least one-third associated with VTEC.

Source
That of causative organism: human or animal, probably bovine in VTEC.

Spread
Foodborne or person to person by faecal–oral route.

Pathogenesis
Damage to vascular endothelium of all organs, readily demonstrable in renal arterioles and glomerular capillaries. No evidence of immune-complex deposition. Acute haemolysis develops during or soon after the prodromal illness. Roles of toxin and immune responses require further elucidation.

Clinical features
- History of preceding diarrhoea or respiratory tract infection.
- Rapidly developing anaemia. Fragmentation and distortion of red blood cells. May be evidence of intravascular haemolysis. Reticulocytosis. Usually mild to moderate thrombocytopenia and moderate leucocytosis.
- Oliguria and uraemia. Oedema. Sometimes hypertension, though unusual. Renal function usually returns to normal within 4 months

though some may progress to chronic renal failure. Outcome unfavourable if dialysis is required for more than 14 days.
- Purpura and bleeding in severe cases.
- Complications include: neurological damage with diffuse or focal lesions; insulin-dependent diabetes; myocardial damage.

Laboratory diagnosis
- Clinical diagnosis confirmed by haematological and biochemical tests.
- Stool culture to determine aetiological agent.

Treatment
- Most patients recover spontaneously so careful management of fluid and electrolyte balance will suffice.
- Dialysis may be required for more severe cases.
- Blood transfusion is seldom necessary.

Prevention

Immediate
- Isolation: enteric precautions.
- Report to health authority so that epidemiological inquiry can be made.
- Identify contacts possibly exposed to same source of infection; search for missed cases; faecal specimens for epidemiological purposes.

Longterm
- Food hygiene to prevent contamination of food vehicles.
- Measures to prevent faecal−oral spread.

Haemophilus influenzae infections

Organism

Haemophilus influenzae: fastidious organism requiring enriched media, speciated by its requirement for V factor (a co-dehydrogenase) and X factor (haemin); the most important human pathogen in the genus *Haemophilus*. Capsulated strains, of which the most invasive is type b, are primary pathogens, common in young children, rare in adults; capsulated strains are typed serologically. Non-capsulated strains are not invasive but cause secondary infections in the respiratory tract. Other species, also carried in the upper respiratory tract, rarely cause disease.

Epidemiology

Distribution

Worldwide common infection; mainly children, frequently symptomless; nasopharyngeal carrier rate in children in USA of non-capsulated *H. influenzae* 60–90% and of type b strains 2–5%. Type b strains commonest cause of bacterial meningitis in North America, less common in Scandinavia and UK, although increase in reported cases in UK during late 1970s and early 1980s from about 300 to 500 per year. Highest incidence aged 6 months to 3 years with a peak in the second 6 months of life; other type b disease, such as epiglottitis and pneumonia, usually children of 18 months to 5 years; boys more often affected than girls; may occur in older children and adults, including elderly.

Source

Human respiratory tract secretions, probably infectious as long as organisms present.

Spread

Close contact; droplets.

Pathogenesis

The virulence of *H. influenzae* type b in young children is due to deficiency of protective antibody. Upper respiratory tract infection may extend rapidly in local tissues, such as the epiglottis or sinuses; infection of the epiglottis associated with gross hyperaemia and

112

oedema. Bloodstream dissemination, e.g. to meninges, can occur at an early stage.

Clinical features
- Nasopharyngitis, often with fever.
- Sinusitis, otitis media (second commonest bacterial cause), laryngitis and pneumonia. In older patients haemophilus is usually secondary invader in chronic bronchitis or after virus infection.
- Acute epiglottitis usually affects children aged 2–5 years, boys 60–70%. Sore throat and fever followed a few hours later by rapid deterioration with respiratory obstruction, collapse and death. Epiglottis fiery-red and swollen. Blood cultures usually positive.
- Bloodstream invasion commonly leads to metastatic infection involving meninges, soft tissues, joints or pericardium.

Meningitis
Prodromal illness with acute respiratory symptoms, sometimes vomiting and diarrhoea. Onset of meningitis usually insidious and difficult to recognize; CSF turbid; no rash.

Cellulitis
Usually involves face.

Arthritis
Usually involves a single large joint, predominantly in children.

Pericarditis
Rare.

Laboratory diagnosis

Primary infections — meningitis
- CSF purulent: small Gram-negative rods, sometimes pleomorphic, usually demonstrable on direct microscopy.
- Culture on appropriate media.
- Countercurrent immunoelectrophoresis of CSF may allow rapid diagnosis.
- Blood cultures should always be taken.

Other sites
- Organism can usually be isolated from site of infection if accessible.
- Blood cultures should be taken.
- Throat swabs should also be cultured.

Secondary (chest) infections
- Direct microscopy of sputum reveals purulence with predominant flora of small Gram-negative rods.
- Isolation from the mixed flora of sputum should be possible using appropriate laboratory methods; the inclusion of dilution cultures aid differentiation between upper respiratory tract colonization and acute bronchitis.

Treatment
- Chloramphenicol first choice in life-threatening infections; ampicillin used for less severe infection but some strains resistant.
- Tracheostomy may be required for severe epiglottitis.
- Aspiration of pus from infected joint.
- Surgical drainage of purulent pericarditis.

Prevention

Immediate
- Isolation: respiratory precautions for meningitis until 24 hours after start of chemotherapy.
- Report to health authority. Meningitis notifiable in UK.
- Contacts: action not generally recommended. Prophylactic chemotherapy with rifampicin for childhood household and nursery contacts has been suggested (p. 185).

Longterm
- Universal immunization of children at 18 months with *H. influenzae* type b polysaccharide vaccine is recommended in USA.

Helminth infections: common intestinal helminths

Threadworm infection *(Enterobius vermicularis)*

Life cycle
Adults live in caecum and adjacent portions of the bowel attached to the mucosa. Gravid female migrates down bowel and emerges from anus at night to lay eggs on the surface of the surrounding skin. Eggs become infective within 2–3 hours and are commonly transferred on fingers to the mouth where they are swallowed and pass down the bowel maturing into adult worms in about 3 weeks.

Distribution
Worldwide, very common infection in young children. Involves households, nursery and primary schools.

Clinical features
May be asymptomatic. Commonly perianal irritation. May invade vagina in women and rarely the peritoneal cavity.

Diagnosis
Adult females may be found on inspection of perianal skin. Eggs detected in swabs taken from perianal skin; not found in faeces.

Treatment
Infection difficult to clear unless all members of family are treated at same time and strict hygiene enforced. Drug treatment should be repeated after 3 weeks: mebendazole single dose 100 mg over age 2 years; or piperazine hydrate or equivalent—up to 2 years 50–75 mg/kg, 2–4 years 750 mg, 5–12 years 1.5 g, over 12 years 2 g daily for 7 days; or pyrantel single dose 10 mg/kg (max. 1 g).

Roundworm infection *(Ascaris lumbricoides)*

Life cycle
Adults in upper small bowel; eggs in faeces non-infectious; infectious embryo develops in soil and is ingested on contaminated vegetables; eggs hatch in small bowel where larvae penetrate mucosa and enter venules or lymphatics; larvae arrested in lungs where they enter the

alveoli and migrate via the bronchi to the gastrointestinal tract and mature into adult forms. Egg to adult about 6 weeks.

Distribution
Worldwide, common in areas with poor sanitation.

Clinical features
Usually asymptomatic. Pneumonitis caused by massive migration of larvae through lungs (Loeffler's syndrome). Heavy infection may result in intestinal obstruction. Migration of adults into bile ducts may cause biliary colic or obstruction.

Diagnosis
Adults may occasionally be passed in stool. Eosinophilia. Unsegmented eggs in stool.

Treatment
- Levamisole first choice: single dose 120–150 mg for adults.
- Also mebendazole 100 mg twice daily for 3 days; pyrantel single dose 10 mg/kg (max. 1 g); piperazine single dose 4 g hydrate or equivalent.

Whipworm infection *(Trichuris trichiura)*

Life cycle
Adults live mainly in the caecum where they attach to the mucosa by their thread-like anterior end. Eggs passed in faeces are not infectious but become embryonated in soil or water. Embryos ingested with food or water and develop into adults within the lumen of the bowel. No invasion and migration through lungs. Cycle takes about 3 months.

Distribution
Common in humid tropics and subtropics.

Clinical features
Mild infections usually asymptomatic. Severe infections may cause chronic diarrhoea, rectal prolapse and anaemia.

Whipworm infection

Diagnosis
Detection of eggs in faeces.

Treatment
- Mebendazole single dose 100 mg over age of 2 years.
- Pyrantel single dose 10 mg/kg (max. 1 g).
- Thiabendazole 25 mg/kg 12-hourly for 3 days in persistent infection.

Hookworm infection *(Ancylostoma duodenale/ Necator americanus)*

Life cycle
Adults attach to mucosa of upper small bowel and suck blood. Eggs passed in faeces to soil where they hatch in 24–48 hours or so releasing rhabditiform larvae. These migrate in the soil and eventually metamorphose into the infective filariform larvae. Larvae of *A. duodenale* usually ingested with food but may penetrate skin; *N. americanus* usually invades through skin. Cycle completed in about 3 months.

Distribution
A. duodenale: southern Europe, northern Africa, southern Asia, Pacific islands, Australasia and restricted areas of South America. *N. americanus*: southern Asia, Pacific islands, central and southern Africa and the Americas.

Clinical features
Mild infection may be asymptomatic especially with *N. americanus*. Heavy infection results in anaemia and hypoproteinaemia.

Diagnosis
Anaemia and eosinophilia. Eggs found in faeces. Speciation by culturing faeces and identifying larvae.

Treatment
- Pyrantel single dose 10 mg/kg (max. 1 g).

- Mebendazole 100 mg twice daily for 3 days.
- Bephenium single dose 2.5 g repeated after 24–48 hours.
- Tetrachloroethylene 2.5–5 ml as suspension.
- Anaemia treated with iron preparation.

Strongyloides infection *(Strongyloides stercoralis)*

Life cycle
Female adults live embedded in the mucosa of upper part of small bowel. Worm has two cycles: parasitic and free-living. Rhabditiform larvae passed in faeces may develop in soil into free-living adults with sexual cycle resulting in eggs, rhabditiform and infective filariform larvae or a direct asexual cycle with progression from rhabditiform larvae to filariform larvae which invade the skin. Rhabditiform larvae in the bowel may develop into filariform larvae and directly invade the bowel wall or perianal skin migrating through the body and eventually maturing in the bowel.

Distribution
Widely distributed in humid tropics and subtropics.

Clinical features
Migration of larvae in the skin may result in cutaneous larva migrans, a linear urticarial eruption, while migration through the lungs may cause a pneumonitis. Immunodepression as a result of disease or therapy may result in overwhelming superinfection with massive invasion of lungs and other organs causing severe illness and even death.

Diagnosis
Eosinophilia. Detection of larvae in faeces or duodenal fluid. Serology: filarial Elisa test cross-reacts with strongyloides.

Treatment
- Thiabendazole, drug of choice: 25 mg/kg 12-hourly for 3 days.
- Mebendazole 100 mg twice daily for 3 days, course of treatment given three times at intervals of 2 weeks.

Schistosomiasis *(Schistosoma mansoni/S. japonicum)*

See p. 66.

Trichiniasis *(Trichinella spiralis)*

Life cycle
When meat containing larval cysts is eaten the larvae are released
into the lumen of the intestine and develop into mature adults within
3–5 days. The females burrow into the bowel wall and give birth to
larvae which are carried in blood and lymph vessels throughout the
body. Those reaching striate muscle eventually encyst and may
remain dormant for a long period until ingested by the next host.

Distribution
Widespread infection of humans derived from pigs, bears, jackals and
wild boar.

Clinical features
Light infection may be asymptomatic. Heavy infection may result in
severe illness or even death. Initial invasion of the bowel wall may
cause diarrhoea, while migration of larvae may result in high fever,
urticarial rashes and circumorbital oedema followed by severe myalgia. Myocarditis is an important cause of death. Once the larvae have
encysted the host reaction subsides usually after a few weeks. When
eventually the larvae die the cysts may calcify and be revealed on
X-ray examination.

Diagnosis
Eosinophilia. Serological tests using Elisa or IFAT may become
positive towards the end of the second week.

Treatment
Careful nursing of severely ill patients and use of corticosteroids to
control host reaction. Thiabendazole and mebendazole appear to be
effective in controlling the intestinal phase but are of doubtful value
against the migrating larvae.

Hepatitis (viral)

Organisms

The main viruses responsible are hepatitis A, B and non-A non-B. None has yet been grown in tissue culture and the agent(s) causing non-A non-B have not been identified. Other viruses causing hepatitis include EB (Epstein–Barr) virus (see p. 140) and cytomegalovirus (see p. 52).

Hepatitis A virus (HAV)

Picornavirus, 27 nm/diameter and agglutinable with convalescent serum and with pooled immunoglobulin, have been demonstrated by electron microscopy in faeces from patients with hepatitis A.

Hepatitis B virus (HBV)

The virus is associated with several particles, antigens and enzymes.
Dane particle (HBV): complex structure with inner core and outer covering, measuring 42 nm diameter.
Surface antigen (HBsAg): amorphous spherical and tubular particles demonstrable in serum during acute infection and in otherwise healthy carriers following subclinical infection. Persistence after acute infection often associated with chronic disease.
Core antigen (HBcAg): confined to hepatocyte.
'e' antigen (HBeAg): nature uncertain, probably derived from HBcAg. Persistence into late convalescence associated with increased risk of chronic disease and high infectivity. Demonstrable in infected haemo-dialysis patients and infrequently in otherwise healthy HBsAg carriers. The latter may also have antibody (antiHBe); some evidence that infectivity is then reduced.
DNA polymerase: associated with HBcAg and HBeAg. Presence related to viral activity.
Delta agent: a defective virus which replicates only in hepatitis B virus infected hepatocytes.

Epidemiology

Distribution

Hepatitis A: worldwide, very common, acute, usually self-limiting infection, especially in areas of poor hygiene and sanitation; often symptomless in children, may be severe in adults. Longterm secular

Epidemiology

changes observed in many countries; substantial decline in Western
Europe and North America 1970s and 1980s with appearance of
proportionately more cases in adults than in children; sometimes
in outbreaks; associated with decline in infection acquired in childhood.

Hepatitis B: worldwide, often chronic infection, high prevalence in
Africa and Asia, where carrier rates of up to 20% in adults have been
reported. In Western countries carrier rates less than 1% in adult
population, 5–10% of adults show evidence of previous infection.
Incidence of disease highest in young adults, particularly homosexuals, i.v. drug abusers, and frequent recipients of blood and blood
products. Higher incidence in health-care workers and laboratory staff
than in general population. In UK about 1000 reported cases per year,
although higher numbers reported in 1983–86 associated with
epidemic in drug abusers. Chronic HBsAg carriage may lead to
chronic hepatitis, cirrhosis and primary hepatic carcinoma, especially
following infections in perinatal period.

Delta hepatitis: worldwide in association with hepatitis B virus
infection, particularly in i.v. drug abusers, in whom outbreaks have
been reported.

Non-A non-B hepatitis: two types described: one resembling hepatitis A, causing waterborne outbreaks mainly reported from India; the
other type (possibly two variants) resembling hepatitis B, giving rise
to post-transfusion hepatitis in many parts of the world.

Source

Hepatitis A: human — virus excreted in urine and faeces for at least a
week before onset of symptoms and for a few days afterwards, and
for a similar length of time in symptomless cases. No carrier state.
Chimpanzees and other primates may be infected, but rarely a source
of human infection.

Hepatitis B: human—blood and body fluids from cases several weeks
before onset and throughout clinical illness; blood and body fluids
from carriers, those with HBeAg most infectious.

Delta hepatitis: human—blood particularly infectious before and
during clinical illness; chronic carriage can occur.

Non-A non-B hepatitis: human.

Spread
Hepatitis A: faecal–oral route, particularly in young children. Food-borne; shellfish harvested from sewage-polluted waters; strawberries contaminated with human slurry; raspberries and other foodstuffs contaminated by excreters. Waterborne.
Hepatitis B and delta hepatitis: close personal contact resulting in blood or body fluid transfer. Sexual contact, particularly homosexual. Unscreened blood and blood products. Contaminated syringes, needles, surgical instruments, tattoo and acupuncture needles and other skin-piercing equipment. Perinatal transmission from carrier mother to infant. Foodborne and faecal–oral transmission not reported.
Non-A non-B hepatitis: hepatitis A type — waterborne, probably faecal–oral spread. Hepatitis B type — blood and blood products.

Pathogenesis — virus B infection

Incubation period
Virion invades hepatocytes and replicates. HBcAg formed in nucleus and HBsAg in cytoplasm. Dane particle and surplus coat released from cell altering cytoplasmic membrane. Virion invades other hepatocytes. HBsAg in circulation 1–3 months after infection and 7 days to 3 months before jaundice. DNA polymerase in circulation soon after infection. HBeAg appears in serum just before jaundice.

Acute hepatitis
Sensitized T cells react with cytoplasmic membrane of infected hepatocytes. Transaminases leak out. Immune complexes of HBsAg and antiHBs deposited in tissues. HBeAg persists in circulation for 1–2 weeks and disappears as antiHBe is formed. AntiHBc appears. Fulminating hepatitis: HBsAg smothered by excess antiHBs.

Recovery
HBsAg disappears after 3 weeks. AntiHBs appears in serum some time later in low titre. Low levels of antiHBc may persist indefinitely. Biliary function recovers first followed by reduction in transaminases.

Clinical features

The incubation period varies with the nature of the infection: virus A about 15—40 days; virus B 2—5 months; epidemic non-A non-B 30—40 days; non-epidemic non-A non-B 45—49 days. It is difficult to distinguish the various forms of hepatitis on clinical grounds. Both virus A and epidemic non-A non-B produce acute self-limiting attacks of hepatitis. Other non-A non-B viruses are generally associated with mild hepatitis but may occasionally result in a fulminating attack. Virus B hepatitis tends to have a longer prodromal period of malaise before jaundice develops and may have prodromal rashes or arthralgia. Delta agent is associated with virus B and may result in acute or chronic hepatitis. Superinfection with delta agent in a carrier of virus B may lead to severe exacerbation of hepatitis.

Acute anicteric hepatitis
- Particularly common in young children.
- Malaise, anorexia, slight diarrhoea and occasional vomiting.
- Enlarged tender liver, increased conjugated bilirubin and transaminase in serum; bilirubin may appear in urine.

Acute icteric hepatitis
- Prodromal period of few days before jaundice appears.
- Anorexia, intense nausea, occasional vomiting, moderate fever in 50%.
- Urine darkens, stools lighten and jaundice appears.
- Liver palpable with smooth tender edge in 70%; splenomegaly in 20%.
- Acute phase in adults lasts for 2—6 weeks; recovery usually complete within 4 months.

Cholestatic hepatitis
- Jaundice deepens rapidly and is associated with marked pruritus.
- Symptoms may persist for 2—6 months but recovery is generally complete.
- Jaundice is of obstructive type; liver biopsy shows histological changes of hepatitis with marked bile stasis.

Clinical features

Fulminant hepatitis
- Typical acute attack progresses to liver failure.
- Deepening jaundice, persistent vomiting, confusion and drowsiness.
- Acute delirium with violent behaviour and occasional fits in children.
- Coma, widespread bleeding, death within 10 days.
- Depth of jaundice and level of transaminases do not closely match severity of liver failure; clotting defects more reliable guide.

Progressive (subacute) hepatitis
- Particularly common in women between 35–40 years of age.
- Initially typical acute attack but illness persists with fluctuating jaundice, mild fever and bouts of vomiting.
- Liver enlarged, splenomegaly develops.
- Liver failure in majority of cases leads to death within 1–3 months.
- Minority survive but with some degree of cirrhosis.

Chronic progressive hepatitis
- Commonly follows acute icteric attack in adult.
- Benign course with slight jaundice, histological changes may persist in liver for many years.
- Outcome generally favourable, very rarely cirrhosis.

Chronic aggressive (active) hepatitis
- Usually follows a subclinical or mild attack, occasionally an acute onset.
- Chronic liver dysfunction, endocrine disturbances, rashes, arthralgia and ulcerative colitis.
- Antinuclear and smooth muscle antibody may be present in serum.
- Extensive necrosis of liver cells and cirrhosis often present.
- Prognosis variable but usually poor.

Laboratory diagnosis

Liver function
Disturbed in all types of acute viral hepatitis. Serum aminotrans-

ferases (SAT) increased. Bilirubin may or may not be raised. Alkaline phosphatase elevated in about 50% of cases.

Hepatitis A
- Peak SAT levels (five to ten times normal) soon after onset of symptoms; gradually fall over 3–4 weeks.
- Detection of antiHAV in serum by radioimmunoassay.
- Demonstration of virus, maximal in faeces in incubation period, not practicable as a routine diagnostic measure; longterm carriage not recognized.

Hepatitis B — acute infection self-limiting
- HBsAg present in serum in late incubation period; may disappear rapidly, more usually persists throughout clinical illness.
- HBeAg detectable in serum during early acute phase just before jaundice and may persist.
- HBcAg not demonstrable in serum, but antiHBc usually present and is thought to indicate replication of HBV in the liver.
- During convalesence HBsAg disappears, liver function tests return to normal, and humoral antiHBs appears; both antiHBc and antiHBs may persist for months or years.

Delta hepatitis
- Detection of IgM antibody response to delta agent.

Hepatitis B — acute infection progressing to chronic disease
- Liver function tests remain abnormal.
- HBsAg persists as may HBeAg, DNA polymerase and antiHBc.

Hepatitis B — subclinical infection
- Detection of HBsAg with or without antiHBc, or detection of anti-HBs in otherwise healthy persons without history of jaundice.
- HBeAg occasionally present, and probably indicates high infectivity; presence of antiHBe apparently associated with reduced infectivity even in presence of HBsAg. Individuals with antiHBc should also be regarded as potentially infectious.
- The risk of eventual chronic liver disease in individuals with HBeAg or antiHBc after subclinical infection not yet determined.

Hepatitis B — carriers
- HBsAg persists in serum but may eventually disappear.
- AntiHBc always present.
- Sometimes HBeAg and increase in polymerase activity.

Methods for detection of antibody vary in sensitivity; radioimmuno-assay and passive haemagglutination most sensitive, complement fixation and immunodiffusion less so.

Treatment
- Rest during the acute phase until the patient feels well.
- Patient allowed to select those foods he finds palatable.
- Corticosteroids reserved for severe subacute or cholestatic hepatitis. Prednisolone 10–20 mg daily until liver function tests have been normal for 4–8 months; then slowly withdrawn.
- Convalescence when patient feels well, urine free from urobilinogen, and serum bilirubin less than 25 mmol/l. Avoid violent exercise for 6 months and alcohol for 1 year.
- Liver failure necessitates urgent admission to specialist unit.
- Antiviral treatment should be considered for patients with evidence of active disease in liver-biopsy specimens, and either HBeAg or hepatitis virus DNA in blood. Various combinations of alpha-interferon, vidarabine, acyclovir and corticosteroids have been used successfully to eliminate the virus.

Prevention

Immediate
- Isolation: enteric/needle precautions.
- Report to health authority; notifiable in UK.
- Identify contacts and search for missed cases, possibly exposed to same source of infection, for epidemiological inquiry.
- Contacts of hepatitis A: household members, sexual contacts and institutional contacts, where faecal–oral spread is likely (e.g. mental handicap units, nurseries), give human normal immunoglobulin (HNIG) as soon as possible after exposure (ineffective after 2 weeks), <10 years 250 mg, 10+ years 500 mg i.m. Not indicated for other contacts.

Prevention

- Food handlers with hepatitis A: HNIG for other food handlers working in same premises. Consider HNIG for persons exposed to food possibly contaminated by infected food handler within 2 weeks of exposure, particularly if food was not cooked after handling or hygienic standards poor.
- Contacts of hepatitis B: exposure to blood or tissue fluids, e.g. needlestick injury, sexual contact, give hepatitis B immunoglobulin (HBIG) 500 iu i.m. within 48 hours. Repeat in 4 weeks or give hepatitis B vaccine if subsequent serological tests show no evidence of past infection and serological status of inoculum is HBeAg positive or not known.
- Infants of hepatitis B carrier mothers, particularly if HBeAg positive or with acute hepatitis B in last 3 months of pregnancy or puerperium: HBIG 100 iu i.m. within 24 hours of birth or exposure, plus hepatitis B vaccine 0.5 ml i.m. in different site; second dose after 1 month, third dose 6 months later. Infants at risk should be determined by serological screening of antenatal women in groups with high prevalence of infection, e.g. Asian ethnic groups.
- Exclude cases of hepatitis A or B from work or school until 7 days after onset of jaundice, or until clinical recovery.
- Exclusion of contacts not justifiable, but non-immune contacts of hepatitis A, who are food handlers, should not directly handle food which is to be consumed without cooking for 5 weeks after contact with index case.

Longterm
Hepatitis A:
- Education to prevent faecal–oral spread, particularly in institutions and nurseries.
- Food hygiene; hygienic production and adequate cooking of shellfish.
- Prophylactic HNIG for travellers to areas outside Europe, North America and Australasia, where hepatitis A is endemic and standards of hygiene poor.
  Short stay up to 2 months: age <10 years 125 mg, 10+ years 250 mg i.m.
  Long stay over 2 months: double these doses.
Serological screening in persons who often travel in these areas.

Prevention

Hepatitis B and delta hepatitis:
- Screening of blood, organ and tissue donors and exclusion of carriers.
- Screening of dialysis patients and staff; isolation of carrier patients and exclusion of carrier staff.
- Sterilization of needles, syringes and other skin-piercing equipment.
- Education of drug-abusers, syringe-exchange schemes.
- Immunization of groups at high risk, such as surgical staff (p. 362).

Herpes simplex infections

Organism
Herpesvirus hominis (herpes simplex): herpes (DNA) virus, morphologically indistinguishable from the varicella zoster virus; grows in various tissue cultures and on chick chorioallantoic membrane. Two serotypes recognized: type 1 implicated in orofacial, skin and neurological infections; type 2 in the genital tract, some cases of aseptic meningitis and radiculitis.

Epidemiology

Distribution
Infection worldwide, very common. Primary infection with type 1 virus usually symptomless in children; between 50% and over 90% of children have antibody by puberty, the proportion depending on social factors. Primary infection with type 2 virus related to sexual activity; may occur without symptoms; infection of neonate during birth may cause severe generalized infection. Genital herpes may be associated with carcinoma of cervix.

Reactivation of primary infection: usually cold sores or genital herpes; generalized infection or persistent local infection is a common manifestation of Aids.

Source
Human. Type 1 usually oral secretions; type 2 usually genital secretions.

Spread
Contact with infected secretions. Type 1 usually by saliva; direct infection of hands may occur in health-care workers. Type 2 usually by sexual contact, including homosexual rectal and oral contact.

Pathogenesis
Virus infects ectoderm and tissues derived from ectoderm forming intranuclear inclusions and giant cells. Primary infections, usually with systemic symptoms, occur in the absence of protective antibody; recurrent infections, following reactivation of latent virus by various non-specific stimuli, common despite high levels of humoral antibody.

129

Clinical features

Primary infection
Often subclinical or mild. Incubation period 2–20 days, usually 4–5 days.
Gingivostomatitis: common manifestation in young children. Sudden onset with high fever, irritability and sore mouth. Typical shallow ulcers with serpiginous edge. General disturbance variable. Sometimes satellite lesions on face, neck or chest; occasionally secondary whitlow. Illness may continue for 2–3 weeks. Adults with stomatitis may be seen by a dentist; constitutional disturbance less severe.
Infection of skin: more frequent in older children and adults. May involve any part of body; lesions above waist usually caused by type 1 virus, below waist by type 2. Herpetic whitlows especially common in nurses, doctors and dentists. Herpetic vulvitis in infants may be dismissed as 'nappy rash'. Patients with eczema very susceptible and may develop eczema herpeticum resulting in severe illness.

Recurrent attacks
Usually involve skin around the mouth or adjacent areas of face; sometimes eye or genital tract. Frequency very variable. Onset heralded by tingling or itching. Papular eruption emerges within few hours and rapidly evolves into cluster of vesicles. After few days these dry to form scabs and eventually heal without permanent scarring. Duration variable, averages 9–10 days.

Eye infection
Primary infection commonest in children and usually takes the form of unilateral follicular conjunctivitis. Recurrent attacks commonest in adults and predominantly involve cornea.

Genital herpes
Caused by type 2 virus in 90–95% of cases. Usually acquired after puberty and transmitted sexually. Clinical illness more common in women; carrier state more common in men.

Nervous system
Herpetic involvement rare; mainly associated with primary infection.

Clinical features

Aseptic meningitis usually caused by type 2 virus; usually follows benign course. Encephalitis commonly caused by type 1 virus; older children and adults; serious condition with high mortality. Diffuse or focal damage in frontotemporal region associated with type 1 virus; myelitis and radiculitis with type 2 virus.

Neonatal infection
Spread from mother's genital tract or from attendant; type 2 virus in 80%. Local lesions overshadowed by catastrophic general disturbance.

Disturbed immunity
Very severe local and generalized infection.

Laboratory diagnosis
● Isolation of virus from vesicle fluid, conjunctival fluid, brain biopsy in human amnion, hamster kidney or other appropriate cell lines; isolation from CSF not usually successful.
● Demonstration of herpesvirus particles in vesicle fluid by electron microscopy (NB morphologically indistinguishable from varicella zoster virus).
● Detection of virus antigen in appropriate specimens by immuno-electrophoresis or fluorescent antibody methods.
● Testing for circulating antibody valuable in primary infection: unhelpful in recurrent infections as pre-existing titre may not change.

Treatment
● Most primary infections mild and settle with palliative treatment.
● Severe local or generalized infections respond to acyclovir; orally, 200−400 mg five times a day for 5 days; or i.v., slow infusion over 1 hour of 5 mg/kg every 8 hours until satisfactory response then orally. Herpes encephalitis 10 mg/kg.
● Eye lesions require expert attention. Usually respond to locally applied acyclovir.
● Prevention of recurrence: acyclovir 200 mg four times a day by mouth or 400 mg twice daily possibly reduced to 200 mg two or three times a day and interrupted every 6−12 months.

Prevention

Immediate
- Isolation: wound precautions for major infection in hospital.
- In hospital inform control-of-infection officer.
- Avoid touching lesions.
- Exclude health-care staff with lesions from working in maternity or neonatal units.
- Caesarean section has been recommended for mothers with genital tract herpes within 2 weeks before expected date of delivery.

Longterm
- General measures to prevent contact spread.
- Chemoprophylaxis for immunocompromised: acyclovir 200–400 mg four times a day by mouth.

HIV infection

Organism
Human immunodeficiency virus (HIV 1): RNA retrovirus isolated in 1983. The virus produces an enzyme, reverse transcriptase, through which the viral genome is copied as DNA then integrated into the host lymphocyte DNA. More recently, another virus has been recognized in West African patients with Aids-like syndrome; this virus, although designated HIV 2, more closely resembles a simian retrovirus.

Epidemiology

Distribution
HIV 1 worldwide. Aids first described in USA 1981. By 1987 major pandemic, nearly 100 000 cases worldwide. Commonest in North and South America, sub-Saharan Africa and western Europe, uncommon in Asia and Far East. Age and sex distribution varies between countries depending on mode of spread. HIV 2 infection reported in West Africa, Portugal, France and Brazil. Apparently similar modes of spread to HIV 1, but disease spectrum not fully defined.

Source
Human. Apparently new viruses, origin obscure but may have evolved from related simian viruses.

Spread
Sexual transmission: homosexual common in North America, western Europe, Australia, giving a male : female ratio of cases about 15 : 1; heterosexual common in sub-Saharan Africa, male : female ratio about 1 : 1.
Parenteral transmission: blood and blood products in countries without donor screening; many haemophiliacs and blood-transfusion recipients infected in North America and Europe before donor screening and heat-treatment of clotting factors in early 1985; may still occur if donation from recently infected person taken before HIV antibody detectable, but risk very small. Transmission by i.m. preparations of Ig and hepatitis B vaccine not reported. Transmission by sharing needles and equipment contaminated by blood gave rise to rapid spread in i.v. drug abusers in eastern USA, southern Europe

and some parts of Scotland. May also be transmitted by re-used, inadequately sterilized surgical equipment and needles or other skin-penetrating instruments. Infection of health-care workers by needle-stick injury and blood splashes reported, but risk small.

Transmission from infected mother to fetus or to infant during or after birth common, extent not yet known, but in mothers with a history of previous transmission up to 65% of infants may be in-fected; breast-milk transmission has been described. Maternal anti-body may persist in infants for up to a year; infection in infants may occur without production of detectable antibody. Prevalence in chil-dren high in areas of spread by i.v. drug abuse.

Transmission by close contact: virus may be present in saliva, tears and other body fluids, but spread not substantiated except by sexual intercourse, blood-to-blood contact and mother to fetus or infant; no evidence of spread by social contact, food, fomites or insects.

Pathogenesis

HIV attaches itself to CD4 antigen on the surface membrane of some cells, particularly helper (T4) lymphocytes but also other cells, no-tably mononuclear and microglial, and enters the cell where the viral genome is incorporated into the host DNA. Infection may remain latent for months or years but probably eventually progresses in a proportion of cases with resultant destruction of helper lymphocytes leading to deficiency of cell-mediated immunity. Thus there is pre-disposition to those diseases (bacterial, fungal, parasitic, viral or neoplastic) normally monitored by cell-mediated immunity. HIV can also affect microglial cells in the brain leading to progressive intel-lectual deterioration and dementia.

Clinical features

Illness of infection

This may develop 1−2 weeks after inoculation of the virus and presents as:

• Infectious mononucleosis-like illness with fever, sore throat, lymph-adenopathy, rash, myalgia and arthralgia.

• Encephalitis.

Clinical features

Seroconversion
Several weeks may elapse before antibodies appear in the blood. In
most people seroconversion is not associated with illness and some
may remain well for several years, perhaps indefinitely. Others may
develop acute aseptic meningitis at the time of seroconversion, or
encephalitis with diffuse or focal signs may appear during the period
of 3 months following conversion. Between 4 and 19% develop Aids
2−5 years after infection, depending on such factors as sexual
behaviour, drug abuse, genetic make-up and place of residence.

Persistent generalized lymphadenopathy syndrome (PGL)
This is defined as lymph node enlargement, with nodes at least 1 cm
in diameter and involving more than one extrainguinal site, with no
obvious cause and persisting for more than 3 months.

Aids-related complex (ARC)
This term is applied to an illness with some of the features of Aids
but lacking the typical opportunistic infections or neoplasia of the
fully developed disease. It is diagnosed when two or more clinical
features accompanied by two or more abnormal laboratory findings
have been present for longer than 3 months.
- Fever 38°C or greater.
- Weight loss 10% or more.
- Persistent generalized lymphadenopathy.
- Diarrhoea either intermittent or persistent.
- Fatigue.
- Night sweats.
- Lymphopenia, neutropenia, thrombocytopenia.
- Anaemia.
- Reduced T-helper lymphocytes.
- Reduced ratio T-helper lymphocytes : T-suppressor lymphocytes.
- Reduced blastogenesis.
- Raised gammaglobulin.
- Cutaneous anergy.

Other conditions associated with persistent HIV infection
- Seborrhoeic dermatitis.
- Hairy leucoplakia.

- Herpes simplex.
- Herpes zoster.
- Impetigo.
- Candidiasis.
- Tinea.

Acquired immune deficiency syndrome (Aids)
The original definition by the Centers for Disease Control in USA
described the syndrome as one in which a person has a reliably
diagnosed disease that is at least moderately indicative of an underlying cellular immune deficiency (such as opportunistic infection or
Kaposi's sarcoma in a person aged less than 60 years) but who at the
time has no other cause of reduced resistance reported to be associated with that disease. This definition has subsequently been modified in the light of detailed knowledge of HIV, and the antigen and
antibody status of the patient taken into consideration (see *Morbidity
and Mortality Weekly Report*, 1987, vol. 36, suppl. 15.)

Opportunistic and other infections
Respiratory tract:
- *Pneumocystis carinii* pneumonia.
- Cytomegalovirus (CMV) infection difficult to assess and often
associated with pneumocystis pneumonia.
- Mycobacterial infection caused by *Mycobacterium xenopi*, *M.
kansasii*, *M. avium intracellulare* and *M. tuberculosis*, often associ-
ated with non-pulmonary lesions.
- Candidiasis of trachea, bronchi and lungs.
- Lymphoid interstitial pneumonia. Pulmonary lymphoid
hyperplasia.
Gastrointestinal tract:
- Diarrhoea of unknown cause.
- Virus infections: herpes simplex, CMV.
- Mycobacterial infections.
- Salmonella infections other than typhoid giving rise to recurrent
septicaemia.
- Protozoal infections: cryptosporidia, isospora, entamoeba.
- Candida.

Clinical features

Nervous system:
- Virus infections: CMV causing encephalitis and retinitis; papovavirus infection.
- Other infections: toxoplasmal and cryptococcal encephalitis.

Tumours
- Kaposi's sarcoma; commonly associated with pneumocystis pneumonia; often disseminated to gastrointestinal tract and elsewhere.
- Lymphoma of brain; other non-Hodgkin's lymphoma of B cell or unknown immunological phenotype.
- Squamous carcinoma of the mouth.
- Cloacogenic carcinoma of rectum.

Disease directly related to HIV infection
- Wasting syndrome (slim disease).
- Encephalitis with dementia and in some cases focal signs.
- Meningitis, myelitis and neuritis.

Laboratory diagnosis
The implications of HIV infection mean that, with very few exceptions, the patient's permission must be obtained before laboratory tests are performed for diagnosis. There must also be facilities for interpretation and discussion of any positive findings with the patients. Patient confidentiality must be protected, possibly by the use of identification codes. Blood should be obtained by venepuncture and great care taken to avoid spillage or 'sharps' injury. Laboratory protocol for identification or management of potentially infective specimens must be observed.

Serology
- *Antibodies* to whole virus and to several virus proteins are detectable in serum (and in other body fluids) between 3 weeks and 3 months after initial infection. False-positive or false-negative results are uncommon in specialist laboratories, but positive reactions should always be confirmed using a different type of test. In the early stages of infection antibodies may be present in low titre, or not demonstrable; follow-up, with repeated testing, is necessary to confirm such infections.

• *Antigens*, especially the core antigen, are detectable in serum for 3–4 weeks after infection until antibody excess supervenes. Detection of antigen in serum at a later stage of infection almost certainly indicates disease progression, but the place of antigen testing in investigation of HIV infection is not yet finalized.

• *Virus isolation* is possible from within lymphocytes even in the presence of high antibody levels; patients with high titres of antibody remain capable, therefore, of transmitting infection.

• *T-lymphocyte subpopulations* (T4 : T8 ratio) are no longer usually estimated for diagnostic purposes.

Treatment
• Counselling and adoption of healthy life style.
• Chemotherapy for opportunistic infections and neoplasms.
• A number of drugs inhibit replication of HIV, most are toxic and none eradicate the virus.
• Zidovudine has proved beneficial in reducing morbidity and prolonging life in patients with Aids or Aids-related complex. It is indicated in patients with Aids, who have recovered from pneumocystis pneumonia within the past 4 months and in patients with multiple infections, weight loss of more than 10%, lymphadenopathy and unexplained fever. Careful haematological monitoring is essential and repeated blood transfusions may be necessary. Dosage: 250 mg by mouth 4-hourly for as long as the drug can be tolerated.

Prevention

Immediate
• Isolation; needle precautions only, unless there is uncontrollable bleeding, severe mental disturbance or readily transmissible secondary infection when appropriate additional precautions should be taken.
• Counselling; safer sexual practices, condoms; self-exclusion from donation of blood, tissues and organs.
• Contacts: counselling as above.
• Report to health authority. Notifiable in many countries. In UK voluntary confidential reports to Communicable Diseases

Surveillance Centre (CDSC) or Communicable Diseases (Scotland) Unit (CD(S)U).
• Exclusion from work or school of HIV-antibody positive persons is not justified, unless there is a complicating secondary infection, e.g. tuberculosis.

Longterm
• Education of persons at risk: avoid penetrating intercourse, particularly rectal; use condoms; avoid sharing injection equipment; avoid pregnancy.
• Education of population on HIV infection and modes of spread. Avoid casual sexual intercourse: avoid injections with unsterile equipment; avoid blood transfusion, if possible, in countries without donor screening.
• Continuing education of health-care staff in laboratory and clinical techniques to avoid injection and other injuries, and to prevent contamination of their skin or mucous membranes with blood or tissue fluids.
• Health-care workers, who are HIV-antibody positive or who are in a recognized risk group for HIV infection, should seek expert advice about their work. Those whose work involves invasive surgical procedures during which injury may occur and their blood come into contact with patient tissues, may need to transfer to other work.
• Self deferral of blood donors; screening of blood, organ and tissue donors. Heat treatment of blood products, and of milk in human-milk banks.
• Routine and pre-travel immunization of HIV-infected persons, with or without symptoms, recommended with live vaccines for measles, mumps, rubella and polio (may excrete virus for long period after vaccination), but not BCG; yellow fever vaccine should not be given to anyone with symptoms from HIV infection. Immunization with inactivated vaccines recommended for pertussis, diphtheria, tetanus, typhoid, cholera and hepatitis B. Vaccine efficacy may be reduced compared with immunocompetent persons. Normal immunoglobulin should be considered after exposure to measles (p. 172) and zoster immunoglobulin after exposure to varicella virus (p. 324).

Infectious mononucleosis

Organism
Epstein–Barr (EB) virus: herpesvirus with an affinity for lymphoid cells, responsible for infectious mononucleosis; the virus is also implicated in Burkitt's lymphoma and nasopharyngeal cancer. Cytomegalovirus infection and toxoplasmosis may present as infectious mononucleosis.

Distribution

Distribution
Worldwide, common, usually symptomless infection in young children. Clinical disease commonest in teenage children and young adults. In UK about 100 new cases per 100 000 consultations in general practice.

Source
Human: pharyngeal secretions.

Spread
Close contact with pharyngeal secretions; kissing.

Pathogenesis
EBvirus is present in B lymphocytes and is capable of transforming lymphocytes in culture; circulating 'atypical' lymphocytes are a constant feature of infectious mononucleosis, but this is a benign disease; the virus remains latent following the acute illness. Maculopapular rash occurs commonly in infectious mononucleosis if ampicillin is prescribed (also talampicillin and amoxycillin); it is probably caused by sensitization to polymers of ampicillin, and is not indicative of allergy to other penicillins.

Clinical features

Incubation period
Uncertain, probably 33–49 days. Clinical presentation variable and syndromes overlap.

Infectious mononucleosis

Clinical features

Juvenile
Lymphadenopathy. Sore throat but seldom exudate. Fever 1–2 weeks.

Adolescent
Vague malaise with low fever. Lymph nodes not prominent.

Anginose
Young adults. Painful congested throat progressing to exudative tonsillitis with patches of white membrane. Palatal petechiae common but not diagnostic. Peritonsillar oedema may cause difficulty in swallowing and breathing. Generalized lymphadenopathy may persist for several months. Splenomegaly and mild hepatitis common; occasionally myocarditis, pericarditis, nephritis, pancreatitis or pneumonitis. Drug-induced rashes very common especially after ampicillin; rubelliform rashes in second week. Fever 2–3 weeks duration.

Prolonged febrile
High fever with severe constitutional disturbance. Usually lymphadenopathy and splenomegaly.

Neurological
Meningitis, encephalomyelitis, polyneuritis or mononeuritis. Considerable overlap. May be sole manifestation. Recovery usually complete but may take many months.

Jaundice
May be presenting feature. Usually mild and subsides rapidly. Evidence of hepatocellular damage. Other features may appear.

Post-viral syndrome
The acute illness may be followed by prolonged debility with lassitude, inability to concentrate and undue fatigue on physical exertion. Most patients recover completely within a few weeks or months; some may remain unwell for 2 or 3 years. There is little to find on clinical examination, though abnormalities may be detected on sophisticated investigation of the immune response to the virus, indicating persistent activity.

Laboratory diagnosis
- Peripheral white cell count and blood film to demonstrate atypical lymphocytes.
- Paul−Bunnell test (or Monospot) should be positive in acute stage, persisting into convalescence; repeat if negative at first. Heterophile antibody tests remain negative in approximately 10% of EBvirus infectious mononucleosis; specific EBvirus antibody may be detected in IgM fraction.
- Liver function tests abnormal in 80% of EBvirus infectious mononucleosis.

Treatment
- Bedrest until temperature settles.
- Analgesics for relief of pain.
- Antibiotics of no value.
- Hydrocortisone i.v. or i.m. for relief of respiratory obstruction followed by prednisolone 10 mg 6-hourly orally for 2 days.
- Convalescence may be protracted and activities may need to be curtailed until recovery takes place.

Prevention
- Isolation: respiratory/wound precautions until diagnosis established.
- General measures to prevent contact with pharyngeal secretions.

Influenza

Organisms

Orthomyxoviruses: approximately 100 nm diameter; ribonucleo-protein core of three antigenic types, A, B and C; virus A responsible for most epidemic influenza; virus B for usually milder infections; virus C probably not a human pathogen.

- Lipid envelope, with projecting haemagglutination sites, surrounds core; haemagglutination sites contain two antigens, H (haemagglutination) and N (neuraminidase).
- Antigenic shift is due to genetic recombination during replication and permits emergence of 'new' virus, in which either or both of H and N antigens are new proteins.
- Antigenic drift results from minor changes within H antigen.
- Virus strain designated according to its type, geographical origin, strain number and year first isolated, e.g. A/Hong Kong/1/68.
- Influenza viruses cultured in chick amniotic cavity and in monkey kidney cell lines; haemagglutination occurs with erythrocytes of various animal species.

Epidemiology

Distribution

Influenza A: worldwide in epidemics associated with antigenic drift of virus; pandemics may follow antigenic shift. The most notable pandemic took place in 1918 following the appearance of the virus now known as swine influenza virus ($HSw N_1$); since the Second World War there have been three pandemics, none of which was as devastating as that following the First World War; in 1947 the A-prime virus appeared ($H_1 N_1$), then 10 years later this was succeeded by the Asian virus ($H_2 N_2$) and again in 1968 by the Hong Kong virus ($H_3 N_2$) causing the last serious outbreak in 1975/76. In 1977 the $H_1 N_1$ subtype reappeared (Red 'flu). Affects all ages; mortality highest in elderly and those with pre-existing cardiac or pulmonary disease. During epidemics in UK, up to 5% population consult their general practitioners; deaths principally in elderly, may exceed 25 000.

Influenza B: worldwide; commonly causes institutional outbreaks in young persons. In USA, association between Reye's syndrome and preceding influenza, particularly B, although this association was not apparent in UK.

Epidemiology

Source
Human: nasal and pharyngeal discharges of cases. Possibly pigs, horses and birds.

Spread
Close contact with discharges of patients; droplets.

Pathogenesis
Virus invades mucosal cells of upper respiratory tract, trachea and bronchi causing destruction of ciliated cells; infection may extend to lungs with resultant necrosis of alveolar epithelium. More commonly, pulmonary infection due to bacterial invasion.

Clinical features

Incubation period
Usually 1–4 days.

Onset
Abrupt, with malaise, headache, shivering, nasal congestion, backache and myalgia especially in adults.

Respiratory symptoms
Sore throat with red glazed pharynx but no exudate. Hacking cough becoming progressively more severe; usually unproductive but over a third of patients cough up plugs of mucopus; chest generally clear. Retrosternal soreness from tracheitis.

Other symptoms
Sweating and dizziness. Nausea, vomiting but no diarrhoea. Eyes suffused and watering; pain on eye movement. Stiffness of neck and back but CSF usually clear.

Convalescence
Fever falls rapidly after 2–5 days. Recovery slow. Post-influenzal depression.

Complications
Bronchitis, bronchiolitis and pneumonia particularly common in elderly. Encephalitis, meningitis and polyneuritis. Reye's syndrome, especially after influenza B.

Laboratory diagnosis

Culture
Nasopharyngeal washings, throat swabs or sputum in monkey kidney cell lines. Typed with specific antisera by haemagglutination-inhibition.

Serology
Complement-fixing antibodies formed against the core antigen, i.e. specific for virus A or virus B but will not distinguish strains. Haemagglutination-inhibiting antibodies formed against infecting strain.

Treatment
- Bedrest in warm room.
- Analgesics for headache and myalgia.
- Codeine or pholcodine for dry cough. Humidification of air.
- Pneumonia during acute phase (generally staphylococcal) — penicillinase-resistant penicillin.
- Post-influenzal pneumonia (usually pneumococcal) — benzyl-penicillin or amoxycillin.
- Oxygen for cyanotic patients.

Prevention

Immediate
- Isolation: respiratory precautions when possible especially with secondary bacterial pneumonia caused by high-grade pathogen.
- General measures to prevent dispersal of infected secretions.
- Amantadine (p. 345).

Longterm
- Inactivated vaccine recommended annually for elderly and those

with chronic heart or lung disease or in patients in whom immuno-suppressive therapy is proposed.

● Routine annual vaccination of healthy persons in closed communities, such as schools, has been advocated but is not generally accepted.

● If epidemic is anticipated vaccination of essential health-care and other staff should be considered. Influenza vaccine, see p. 363.

Kawasaki disease (mucocutaneous lymph node syndrome)

Organism
Believed to be infectious but organism not identified.

Epidemiology

Distribution
First described in Japan in late 1960s and since reported from many other countries; most cases under 5 years of age. Mainly sporadic but outbreaks have been reported. In UK about 100 cases per year reported.

Source
Not known.

Spread
Not known.

Pathogenesis
Widespread angiitis with surrounding acute inflammation, at some sites progressing to fibrinoid necrosis. Angiitis of coronary vessels may result in aneurysm and thrombosis. Carditis is common finding and main cause of death. Thrombocytosis may be pronounced during the second and third weeks of illness and predispose to thrombosis.

Clinical features
The diagnosis is established clinically when five out of the following six criteria have been met:
- *Fever of unknown aetiology*: lasting for 5 days or longer and unresponsive to antibiotics.
- *Conjunctivitis*: usually bilateral; bulbar surfaces more severely affected.
- *Lips and mouth*: lips dry with redness and fissuring; tongue has strawberry appearance; oropharynx diffusely inflamed.
- *Periphery of limbs*: early stage — redness of palms and soles with accompanying oedema of dorsum of hands and feet; late stage — membranous desquamation beginning around finger tips.
- *Exanthem*: pleomorphic rash, most prominent on trunk; absence of vesicles and crusts.

- *Lymphadenopathy*: acute non-suppurative enlargement of cervical lymph nodes.
- Additional features include: coronary artery thrombosis, hydrops of gallbladder, meningitis, arthritis, urethritis and otitis media.
- Prognosis is worst in boys under 1 year of age with prolonged fever and a rash accompanied by a very high ESR.

Laboratory diagnosis
Diagnosis based on clinical assessment.

Treatment
- Aspirin 30−50 mg/kg a day during acute phase.
- Echocardiography for detection of coronary artery aneurysm. If present after 30 days continue with aspirin 10 mg/kg daily until it resolves.
- Gammaglobulin in high dosage i.v. has been reported to be beneficial.

Prevention

Immediate
- Isolation: unnecessary once diagnosis has been established.
- Report clusters of cases to health authority for epidemiological investigation.
- In UK, paediatricians should report cases to the British Paediatric Surveillance Unit.

Longterm
- None.

Legionella infection

1 Legionnaires disease

Organism
Legionella pneumophila (six serotypes): flagellated Gram-negative rod having fastidious *in vitro* growth requirements; first isolated in yolk sac of embryonated hen's egg; grows within human embryonic lung fibroblasts in tissue culture; endotoxin production demonstrable. Other *Legionella* spp. recently described also associated with pneumonia.

Epidemiology

Distribution
First recognized in an outbreak of pneumonia in Philadelphia, USA in 1976; evidence of infection at least as early as 1940s. Infection probably worldwide; endemic and in common source outbreaks; uncommon cause of pneumonia (legionnaires disease) and rare non-pneumonic respiratory disease (Pontiac fever). Incidence of legionnaires disease highest in late summer and autumn; accounts for less than 5% of community-acquired pneumonias except during outbreaks. Affects mainly middle-aged and elderly, especially males, and those with a history of smoking or pre-existing disease. In UK about 200 cases reported annually with case fatality of about 10%; nearly one-third of cases infected overseas.

Source
Aqueous environment: outbreaks associated with domestic hot water systems in large buildings; with water-cooling systems of air-conditioning plants and in industrial processes; with whirlpool spas and with respiratory therapy equipment.

Spread
Airborne: inhalation of droplets or droplet nuclei. No convincing evidence of person-to-person spread.

Pathogenesis
In fatal cases acute fibrinopurulent pneumonia affecting one or more lobes; relatively little interstitial involvement, but with evidence of

spread to larger bronchioles and to pleura; extension to lymphatics and haematogenous spread. Organisms also demonstrated in liver and spleen. Lung biopsies have revealed fibrinopurulent pneumonia or organizing pneumonia with interstitial fibrosis.

Clinical features

Incubation period
Usually 2–10 days, up to 18 days.

Onset
Slight rise in temperature, malaise, headache and widespread myalgia. Progressively more ill with shivering and temperature rising to 40+°C. Relative bradycardia in 50%. Diarrhoea often an early feature.

Respiratory symptoms and signs
Coryza or sore throat followed by dry cough, becoming productive with clear mucoid or purulent sputum. Sputum blood-streaked in 20–40%. Pleuritic pain in 30%. Early, few inspiratory crepitations; later, signs of consolidation.

Course
Reaches peak after 4–5 days. Severely ill with continuous high fever. Marked prostration. Mental confusion in 50%. Illness abates after 8–10 days. Slow convalescence and persistent radiological changes.

Radiological changes
Not characteristic. Consolidation tends to spread to other lung. Changes may persist for several months. Large effusions in patients receiving corticosteroid therapy. Cavitation uncommon.

Complications
Respiratory, circulatory or renal failure.

Laboratory diagnosis
● Moderate leucocytosis with left shift, sometimes lymphopenia, elevated ESR.
● Proteinuria, occasional haematuria.

Laboratory diagnosis

- Hyponatraemia, elevated aminotransferases and hypoalbuminaemia.
- Isolation of the organism from bronchial or transtracheal aspirate, or lung biopsy, is more successful than from sputum and requires special media containing cysteine and iron (Greave's medium or charcoal yeast-extract agar).
- Serum antibody detection, by indirect fluorescent-antibody technique, basis of most diagnoses. Antibodies usually apparent from about tenth day of illness, occasionally appearance delayed into convalescence. At least a fourfold rise in titre should be demonstrated; a single titre of 1/128 is acceptable if the clinical syndrome is characteristic. Elisa and countercurrent immunoelectrophoretic methods have also been described.
- Demonstration of the bacterium by direct fluorescent-antibody staining of sputum, lung biopsy or post-mortem lung may be more satisfactory.

Treatment

- Erythromycin: adults 0.5–1.0 g 6-hourly orally or 2–4 g i.v. daily; children 15 mg/kg 6-hourly orally.
- Rifampicin in addition if response unsatisfactory.
- Oxygen or mechanical ventilation for respiratory failure.
- Dialysis for renal failure.

Prevention

Immediate

- Isolation: unnecessary once diagnosis has been established.
- Report to health authority to enable local epidemiological investigation.
- Report also to national health authority, especially if travel associated, so that related cases can be identified.
- Search for cases possibly exposed to same source of infection.
- Bacteriological examination and early treatment of water systems implicated epidemiologically in outbreaks of disease.
- Bacteriological examination of water systems associated with sporadic cases not usually justified, except in possible nosocomial infections and infections with rare serogroups of *L. pneumophila* or other species of legionella.

Longterm
- Design of water systems in buildings to store hot water at not less than 60°C and deliver it at not less than 50°C and to store and deliver cold water at not more than 20°C. The design of hot water systems should also ensure that stagnation of water in peripheral parts of the systems is avoided.
- Design of air-conditioning systems using air-cooled rather than water-cooled condensers.
- Careful maintenance and hygiene of air-conditioning systems and water supplies to ensure the above quoted temperatures, and to prevent growth of legionella in existing water-cooled air-conditioning systems. This should include biennial cleaning of calorifiers (heating cylinders) so that all debris and sediment is removed.
- Use of distilled water in medical humidifiers and nebulizers, and thorough cleaning following each period of use of equipment.
- Frequent cleaning and water changes of whirlpool spas and continuous disinfection.
- Routine testing of water systems for legionella is not recommended.

2 Pontiac fever

Pontiac fever is also caused by *L. pneumophila* and has affected people working on condensers of air-conditioning plants and bathers in whirlpool spas. It differs clinically from legionnaires disease in having a shorter incubation period of 5−66 hours (median 36−37 hours), a much shorter benign course of 2−5 days and absence of pneumonia.

Leptospirosis

Organisms
Spirochaetes: two main species — *Leptospira interrogans*, which includes the majority of pathogens, and, *L. biflexa*; both include many serotypes (serovars), some pathogenic and others saprophytic. Identification of serovars requires characterization of genus, group and type-specific antigens. Those most prevalent in the UK are *L. icterohaemorrhagiae, L. canicola* and *L. hebdomadis*.

Epidemiology

Distribution
Worldwide zoonosis, most common in males and usually occupationally acquired. In UK about 80 reported cases per year in 1980s; seasonal peak in summer and autumn: 1−5 deaths per year. *L. icterohaemorrhagiae* causes the most severe disease (Weil's disease) and is usually associated with exposure to rats' urine in sewermen, miners, fish workers, fish farmers and agricultural workers in rice fields. May occur in participants in water sports, such as canoeing and wind surfing on polluted inland lakes and rivers, and in swimmers in these waters. *L. hebdomadis* infection is associated with cattle farming; increased in many countries in 1970s and 1980s following an increase in size of cattle herds and the adoption of the herring-bone milking parlour system, which exposes workers more readily to splashing with cow's urine. *L. canicola* infection is associated with handling dogs.

Source
Urine of infected rodents, dogs and farm animals. Carrier animals may excrete the organism for long periods of time.

Spread
Direct contact of skin, especially if abraded, mucous membranes or conjunctiva with infected urine, or water or soil polluted by infected urine. Organisms survive for several months in moist alkaline environment. Water- and foodborne outbreaks have been reported. Person-to-person transmission has not been described.

Pathogenesis

Infection is through mucous membranes, conjunctivae or abraded skin; bacteraemia follows at the end of the incubation period; invasion of liver, kidney, lung, meninges and the eye may follow; 'septic shock' occurs in severe infections.

Clinical features of leptospirosis

The severity varies with the serovar from a mild febrile illness to a fatal attack characterized by severe jaundice, haemorrhage and renal failure.

Incubation period

Commonly 7 – 12 days but may extend from 4 to 19 days.

Clinical features of Weil's disease

Onset

Sudden 62%; gradual 38% becoming rapidly worse on fourth or fifth day.

First week

Rigors and shivering; fever; malaise and severe debility; headache and myalgia; nausea, vomiting, abdominal pain and haematemesis; jaundice; skin haemorrhages; injected eyes.

Second week

Jaundice deepens; haemorrhages; iritis, optic neuritis; meningitis and encephalitis; renal failure. Most deaths occur at this stage.

Third week

Illness abates. Relapse in 32%. Slow recovery over 6 – 12 weeks.

Clinical features of canicola fever

Onset

Sudden with shivering or rigors. Intense headache.

Clinical features of canicola fever

Other symptoms
- Fever; prostration; myalgia; nausea, slight vomiting; occasional mild jaundice.
- Neck stiffness and muscle weakness common presentation. CSF shows lymphocytosis and increased protein.
- Conjunctival injection in 50% of cases. Fleeting erythematous rashes.
- Urine contains protein and few casts; seldom renal failure.
- Acute stage subsides after 10–14 days. Slow convalescence. Recovery complete.

Clinical features of other forms of leptospirosis
Leptospirosis should be considered in patients with unexplained fever, jaundice or meningitis, especially when accompanied by conjunctival suffusion and a polymorphonuclear leucocytosis.

Laboratory diagnosis
- Demonstration of leptospires by dark-ground illumination of blood or fresh alkaline urine, but experience is required to avoid confusion with artefacts.
- Culture of blood (first week of illness) and fresh urine (second and subsequent weeks) in appropriate fluid medium or by intraperitoneal inoculation of a guinea pig; urine for culture should be alkaline, and potassium citrate may be prescribed to achieve this.
- Detection of antibodies, rising in titre from the second week, by agglutination, complement fixation, immunofluorescence or other methods, is the chief means of diagnosis; examination of serum during convalescence may be necessary to determine the infecting serovar as some antibodies appear relatively late; antibody usually persists long after recovery.
- Lymphocytic response is found in the CSF of patients with leptospiral meningitis.
- Polymorphonuclear leucocytosis and albuminuria are common. Blood urea may be raised; aminotransferases may be normal or raised.

Treatment
- Antibiotics of doubtful value when given early and of no apparent

Treatment

---

value when given in advanced cases. Optimum choice — benzyl-penicillin or tetracycline.
- Dialysis for renal failure.
- Blood transfusion for severe haemorrhage.

Prevention

Immediate
- Isolation: respiratory/enteric precautions until diagnosis has been established.
- Report to health authority; notifiable in UK.
- Investigate exposure to animals and contaminated inland waters.

Longterm
- Protective clothing to prevent occupational exposure.
- Rodent control.
- Hygiene in the fish industry and fish farming.
- Avoidance of contact with known polluted inland lakes and rivers.

Listeriosis

Organism
Listeria monocytogenes: aerobic, Gram-positive rod, resembling *Corynebacterium* spp. with which it may be confused; the chief differentiating feature of *L. monocytogenes* is its tumbling motility at 18–20°C. Infection induces monocytosis in experimental animals; polymorphonuclear leucocytosis usual in man.

Epidemiology

Distribution
Worldwide uncommon infection; usually sporadic, occasionally foodborne outbreaks reported. Occurs most often during pregnancy, in the very young, the elderly or immunocompromised, but about one-third cases in UK are seen in previously healthy young adults. May cause abortion. An important cause of neonatal septicaemia and meningitis. Cutaneous infection reported in veterinarians. Incidence appears to be increasing in Europe and North America; in UK over 250 cases 1987, with peak in late summer and early autumn.

Source
Widespread infection in domestic and wild animals, and in environment. Increase of infection in farm animals, particularly sheep in UK, has been associated with feeding of silage.

Spread
Foodborne outbreaks have been reported associated with contaminated raw cabbage, milk and cheese. Mother to fetus *in utero* or during passage through infected birth canal. Direct contact with infected animals. Case-to-case spread in nurseries has been reported.

Pathogenesis
Infection occurs most commonly in neonates, the elderly or debilitated, or the immunocompromised; pathogenesis is ill-understood.

Fetal infection associated with widespread areas of focal necrosis, including the placenta; mononuclear infiltration of necrotic areas. Similar histology reported in rare fatal adult cases.

Clinical features

Pregnant women
Mild febrile illness with low-grade bacteraemia. Rapid recovery during puerperium. Persistent infection may cause habitual abortion.

Fetus and neonate
Heavy maternal infection results in overwhelming septicaemia. Light maternal infection accompanied by septic meningitis within 3 weeks of birth (see pp. 45 and 179).

Septicaemia
In healthy adults, or an opportunistic infection in immunodeficient. May culminate in septic meningitis.

Septic meningitis
Newborn and adults over 40 years.

Other syndromes
Oculoglandular, anginose with negative Paul–Bunnell test, pneumonia, urethritis in men, papular or pustular rash in veterinarians, and purulent conjunctivitis in poultry workers.

Laboratory diagnosis

Neonate
L. monocytogenes can be isolated from meconium, skin papules, purulent conjunctival discharge, blood cultures or CSF.

Adult — meningitis
- CSF: initially neutrophil response, later lymphocytic; intracellular or extracellular Gram-positive rods; culture.
- Blood cultures may be positive especially early in disease.
- Blood polymorphonuclear leucocytosis.

Adult — other syndromes
Culture of *L. monocytogenes* from suitable specimens should be

possible if laboratory is alerted. Selective media, or other methods, are usually necessary to isolate from sites with mixed flora.

Treatment
- Determine sensitivity of infecting strain as quickly as possible.
- Tetracycline is drug of choice for most infections.
- Chloramphenicol choice for meningitis.
- Treat for at least 10 days to prevent relapse.

Prevention

Immediate
- Isolation: enteric/wound precautions in maternity unit.
- Ampicillin prophylaxis should be considered for newborn from infected mothers.
- Report to health authority; meningitis notifiable in UK.
- Search for possible associated cases and investigation of likely common sources of infection.

Longterm
- Pregnant women should avoid contact with infected animals.
- Care by veterinarians and farmers in handling aborting animals and fetuses.
- Pasteurization and careful hygienic production of milk, cheese and other dairy products.

Lyme disease

Organism
Borrelia burgdorferi: Gram-negative, microaerophilic spirochaete.

Epidemiology

Distribution
Lyme arthritis first described in Old Lyme, Connecticut, USA in 1975; since reported in most eastern states of USA, in Europe and Australia. Arthritis unusual in Europe, where erythema chronicum migrans, the primary skin manifestation, was first recognized in Sweden in 1909; common in forested areas, such as southern Sweden and Austria. In UK erythema chronicum migrans reported in Scotland, Thetford forest in East Anglia and New Forest in Hampshire; mostly in summer months; appears uncommon.

Source
Deer, possibly dogs and other domestic animals, wild rodents.

Spread
Tick-borne: *Ixodes ricinus* in Europe; *I. dammini* in USA. Not transmissible from person to person.

Pathogenesis
Not elucidated. In the early stage of infection the organism is widely distributed and can be demonstrated in skin lesions, blood and sometimes CSF. Immunological responses contribute to the later manifestations. Coincidence of severe disease and certain histocompatibility antigens has been reported.

Clinical features
The clinical classification of Lyme disease into three stages has proved unsatisfactory because of variability in presentation and evolution. It has been found to be more practical to regard the different manifestations as early and late.

Early
- Local lesion at site of tick bite.
- Lymphadenitis: single or multiple.

Lyme disease

- Low-grade fever with nausea, vomiting, headache, myalgia and arthralgia.
- Erythema chronicum migrans may appear about 5 weeks after infection and spread slowly over a period of several months. Present in about 7% of those infected.

Late

- Nervous system: chronic meningitis, meningoencephalitis, cranial nerve palsies, transverse myelitis, radicular pain and peripheral neuropathy.
- Heart: arrythmias may be severe and warrant use of pacemaker; myocarditis and pericarditis.
- Joints: arthritis developing months or years after initial infection. Children usually have one joint affected; adults more than one with high incidence of recurrent attacks.
- Skin: acrodermatitis chronica atrophicans, lymphadenitis benigna cutis.

Laboratory diagnosis

Serology

Except in very early disease antibody is detectable in serum and CSF by immunofluorescence and Elisa methods. False-positive reactions may occur in systemic lupus erythematosis and in syphilis.

Culture

Not a routine diagnostic method, but *B. burgdorferi* can be grown on appropriate media.

Treatment

- Benzylpenicillin for 10 days.
- Cefotaxime or ceftriaxone when CNS is affected.

Prevention

Immediate

- Isolation unnecessary once diagnosis is established.
- Report to health authority. Not notifiable in UK, unless presenting with aseptic meningitis.

Lyme disease

Prevention

- Investigate possible source of infection.
- Search for missed cases so that treatment may be offered.

Longterm
- Education on mode of transmission of the disease.
- Clothing to prevent tick bites in infested areas.
- Tick control on domestic animals and pets.

Malaria

Organisms
Parasites of the genus *Plasmodium*; man is the intermediate host for four species, *P. vivax*, *P. falciparum*, *P. malariae* and *P. ovale*; female anopheline mosquito is the definitive host.

Epidemiology

Distribution
Widespread in tropics and subtropics; resurgence in many countries in late 1970s and 1980s following failure of malarial eradication programmes. Benign tertian (*P. vivax*) common in Indian subcontinent, South East Asia and Central America; *P. ovale* mainly in West Africa. Malignant tertian (*P. falciparum*) common in Africa, South America and South East Asia; chloroquine-resistant strains widespread in latter two regions and in East Africa. Quartan (*P. malariae*) mainly Africa.

Probably about 100 million cases and 1 million deaths annually worldwide. Increasing imported disease in North West Europe; in UK over 2000 cases per year in mid-1980s, with 5–10 deaths per year due to *P. falciparum* malaria in persons who had not taken prophylaxis. A few indigenous cases of *P. falciparum* have been reported associated with international airports in Europe, due to infected mosquitoes carried in aircraft from Africa. Occasional reports of transfusion-associated cases.

Source
Human only. Non-human primates are infected with plasmodia of different species but transmission to humans rarely occurs.

Spread
Bite of infected female anopheline mosquito; usually bite at dusk or dawn; some anopheline mosquitoes are more effective than others in transmitting malaria. Blood transfusion or bone marrow transplant from infected donors. Syringes and needles contaminated with infected blood in i.v. drug abusers and accidental inoculation in health-care workers. Mother to fetus in congenital malaria.

Pathogenesis

Pre-erythrocyte stage
Sporozoites, produced following sexual cycle in mosquito, introduced
by mosquito bite; incubation period corresponds to pre-erythrocyte
stage when organism multiplies asexually in the liver; merozoites
formed which either infect other liver cells and repeat the exo-
erythrocytic cycle, or enter red blood cells.

Erythrocyte stage
Within erythrocytes merozoites develop into trophozoites, which
mature into schizonts and segment forming further merozoites;
erythrocytic cycle repeated and rupture of erythrocytes later tends to
become synchronous, accounting for periodicity of fever. Some
trophozoites eventually form gametocytes which require re-entry into
the mosquito for further development. Cell debris and malarial pig-
ments are taken up by reticuloendothelial system, leading to hepatosplenomegaly. In falciparum malaria especially, erythrocytes sludge
blocking small blood vessels in brain and other organs; this and
associated immune reaction are responsible for many of the clinical
features.

Sickle-cell trait associated with relative resistance to malaria. Red
blood cells lacking Duffy antigen are unsuitable for attachment of *P.
vivax*.

Clinical features
● Incubation period usually 10–15 days. Sometimes prolonged to 4
weeks in quartan malaria or even longer with some strains of *P.
vivax*.
● Primary attacks in non-immunes tend to have abrupt onset and
severe course. Some days may elapse before periodic fever is
established.
● Recurrent attacks in semi-immunes tend to be mild and a brief
interlude in chronic debilitating disease. Periodic fever from beginning.
● Periodic fever with peak every 48 hours in tertian and 72 hours in
quartan; may remain irregular in malignant malaria.
● *Cold stage*: rigor, vomiting, skin cold and blue, temperature rises,
convulsions in children; duration 1–2 hours.

Clinical features

- *Hot stage*: skin dry and hot, intense throbbing headache, high fever, restlessness merging into delirium and light coma; duration 2–6 hours.
- *Sweating stage*: profuse sweating, rapid drop in temperature, patient exhausted but feeling much better; duration 2–4 hours, sleep follows.
- *Common symptoms*: malaise, headache, anorexia, nausea, vomiting, joint pains.
- *Common signs*: splenomegaly, hepatomegaly, anaemia and jaundice.

Vivax malaria
Serious complications rare, seldom fatal. Jaundice uncommon, anaemia mild. Untreated vivax malaria becomes quiescent after 2 months or so.

Falciparum malaria
Difficult to diagnose and exceedingly treacherous in non-immunes. Fever may be completely irregular. Anaemia is a prominent feature. Specific organs may bear brunt of damage: brain, gastrointestinal tract, liver, kidneys, cardiovascular and haemopoietic systems. Blackwater fever in sensitized individuals. Falciparum malaria in semi-immunes causes mild illness with low mortality.

Ovale malaria
Usually part of mixed infection. Course similar to vivax.

Quartan malaria (P. malariae)
Insidious onset. Regular periodicity established early. Course similar to vivax. Cerebral disturbance prominent. Renowned for chronicity and relapses. Nephrosis may develop in children with persistent infection. This differs from the nephrotic syndrome of children in temperate climates in that it occurs at a later age (3–5 years), responds less well to corticosteroids and has a worse prognosis. It does not respond to antimalarial therapy. Quartan malaria also associated with tropical splenomegaly syndrome.

Laboratory diagnosis
- Confirmation by demonstration of plasmodia in either thick or thin blood smears is essential; the various *Plasmodium* spp. are differentiated morphologically; mixed infections occur occasionally.
- If an experienced pathologist is not available for a patient with severe symptoms, blood must be taken without delay and treatment started immediately before results are known.
- Parasitaemia may be difficult to demonstrate in patients who have taken inadequate prophylaxis in quartan malaria and in falciparum malaria especially with gross haemolysis.
- Serology: IFAT may be helpful in retrospective diagnosis, recurrent fever and in tropical splenomegaly syndrome.

Treatment — uncomplicated malaria in non-immunes

Strain sensitive
Chloroquine base 600 mg (4 tablets) orally followed by 300 mg after 6 hours, then 300 mg daily for 2 days.

Strain resistant
Quinine dihydrochloride or bisulphate 600 mg (2 tablets) orally every 8 hours for at least six doses, then a single oral dose of pyrimethamine 75 mg and sulphadoxine 1.5 g (Fansidar 3 tablets). When Fansidar resistance is present a combination of quinine and tetracycline may prove effective. With multiresistant strains mefloquine should be considered, if available.

Treatment — uncomplicated falciparum malaria in semi-immunes

Strain sensitive
Chloroquine 600 mg orally.

Strain resistant
Pyrimethamine 50 mg and sulphadoxone 1 g orally.

Treatment — complicated falciparum malaria

Strain sensitive
Quinine by i.v. infusion over 4 hours in a dose of 5–10 mg/kg base. The total dose should not exceed 500 mg at one time and treatment should be given at intervals of 12–24 hours until oral therapy is feasible. When the plasmodium is more resistant a higher dosage may be necessary (16.7 mg/kg in 4 hours by i.v. infusion followed by 8.4 mg/kg in 4 hours every 8 hours). After 48 hours reduce dose and continue for further 5 days. Quinine should not be given i.v. to infants but may be given i.m. in a dose not exceeding 5 mg/kg. Follow quinine with standard oral course of chloroquine. Chloroquine base 200 mg i.v. every 12 hours may be used as an alternative to quinine.

Strain resistant
Intravenous quinine followed by quinine orally for 3–5 days, then a final dose of 3 tablets of Fansidar.

Additional therapy and management
- Careful supervision of fluid balance to prevent pulmonary oedema.
- Monitor blood glucose to detect and treat hypoglycaemia.
- Diagnose and treat secondary septicaemia in algid malaria.
- Correct anaemia by blood transfusion if necessary.
- Peritoneal or haemodialysis in renal failure.

Treatment — other forms of malaria
- Acute attacks: chloroquine as for uncomplicated falciparum malaria.
- Eradicate exo-erythrocytic phase of *P. vivax* and *P. ovale* with primaquine 7.5 mg twice daily or pamaquine 8–10 mg of base thrice daily by mouth for 14–21 days. If severe deficiency of glucose-6-phosphate dehydrogenase do not give 8-aminoquinolines but use instead suppressive treatment with chloroquine for 2–3 years. Similarly these drugs should not be used during pregnancy but suppressive treatment with chloroquine should be prescribed until the baby is born, whereupon the mother should be offered curative treatment with primaquine or pamaquine.

Prevention

Immediate
- Isolation: unnecessary once diagnosis has been established.
- Report to health authority; notifiable in UK.
- In non-malarious areas, investigate source of infection.
- In endemic areas, identify localities with high levels of infection so that mosquito-control measures may be applied.

Longterm
- Personal protection by clothing to cover limbs between dusk and dawn; application of insect repellent to uncovered skin; sleeping under mosquito nets.
- Chemoprophylaxis for travellers to endemic areas provides relative protection. Begin a week before arrival in area and continue for at least 4 weeks after leaving. Recommended drugs in 1988:

   North Africa and Middle East: chloroquine 300 mg weekly or proguanil 200 mg daily for adults.

   Asia, China, Africa (East, Central and West), Central and South America and Oceania: chloroquine 300 mg weekly plus proguanil 200 mg daily for adults.

   Dosage for children: under 1 year, one-quarter adult dosage, 1–5 years, one-half adult dosage, 6–12 years, three-quarters adult dosage, and over 12 years, adult dosage.

   Hyperendemic areas: where there is a high incidence of multiple-resistant *P. falciparum* malaria, sulphonamide plus pyrimethamine is very effective but toxic.

In the event of fever in an area where diagnostic facilities are lacking, three Fansidar tablets should be taken immediately to abort breakthrough of the parasite.
- Advice on prophylaxis updated in WHO *Weekly Epidemiological Record*. In UK occasional reports in Public Health Laboratory Service (PHLS) *Communicable Disease Report*. Telephone advice: Birmingham 021–772 4311, Glasgow 041–946 7120 (ext 247), Liverpool 051–708 9393, London 01–636 8636 (ext 212), 01–636 7921 (recorded message).
- Blood donors: exclude donations from transfusion (may be used for plasma fractionation) for at least 6 months after returning from

endemic area, unless screened and shown to be free from malarial antibodies.

- In endemic areas: elimination of mosquito-breeding areas; living accommodation should be screened; spray accommodation with residual insecticide; personal protective measures; chemoprophylaxis; early and effective treatment of cases.

Measles

Organism

Measles virus: paramyxovirus (RNA), approximately 140 nm in diameter; one serotype. Grows in several tissue culture cell lines typically forming syncytium of multinucleated giant cells with intra-nuclear inclusions.

Epidemiology

Distribution

Universal disease; symptomless infection very uncommon. Endemic in large communities with epidemics in alternate years; in small isolated populations endemic disease is not sustained and extensive epidemics follow reintroduction of infection after a long interval; seasonal peak in early spring in temperate climates.

Highest incidence in pre-school children; rare in infants because of maternal passive immunity. In North America routine immunization of children has reduced incidence by 99%; now more common in young adults; sometimes an imported infection. In UK a smaller reduction of about two-thirds achieved because of lower vaccine acceptance; only 70% children immunized by age of 2 years.

Severe disease in poorly nourished children in tropical countries where mortality rates of 10% or more reported; severe, often fatal measles pneumonia may occur in immunocompromised; more serious disease in adults than children.

Subacute sclerosing panencephalitis (SSPE) follows measles in 5–10 per milion cases at median interval of about 7 years after infec-tion; median age of onset of SSPE 10 years; commoner in males than females. Incidence declined in North America following successful measles vaccination programme and appears to be falling in UK.

Source

Human. Respiratory secretions of case; most infectious during pro-dromal illness; infectivity ceases within a few days of onset of rash.

Spread

Droplet or contact with respiratory secretions. Very infectious.

Pathogenesis

Entry
Via the respiratory tract; multinucleate giant cells in nasal secretions during prodromal period; viraemia follows; in fatal cases widespread dissemination of virus demonstrable.

Post-infectious encephalitis
Probably an abnormal immune response; in fatal cases demyelination and perivascular cellular infiltration. Virus not recoverable from CSF.

Subacute sclerosing panencephalitis
An active infection: high titres of IgM and IgG measles antibody in serum and CSF. In fatal cases intranuclear inclusions and sometimes syncytium formation in brain cells; virus can also be isolated from brain.

Clinical features

Incubation period
Usually 10–14 days.

Prodromal period
Commonly 3–4 days but may extend to 8 days. Fever. Irritability, drowsiness, sometimes convulsions in young children. Respiratory tract catarrh and conjunctivitis. Koplik's spots on mucous membranes pathognomonic. Occasionally prodromal erythematous rashes. Lymph nodes enlarged.

Exanthem
Rash appears on back of neck and face, evolves from above downwards and consists of dusky-red maculopapules. Individual lesions coalesce to form blotches. Koplik's spots disappear as rash emerges. After 48 hours the erythema fades to leave pigmentation called staining. Temperature returns to normal as rash reaches staining stage. Fine desquamation after severe rash. Acute illness lasts 7–10 days.

Complications
Laryngeal obstruction, otitis media and bronchopneumonia. Appendicitis. Post-infectious encephalitis and, rarely, SSPE.

Laboratory diagnosis
Rarely necessary.

Serology
Neutralizing, haemagglutination-inhibiting and complement-fixing antibodies detectable soon after appearance of rash, fall gradually after recovery but persist in low titre indefinitely. Virus isolation from throat washings.

Treatment
- Nurse in warm room.
- Simple analgesics for relief of headache and backache.
- Sedative cough linctus or humidification of air.
- Antibiotics not required for uncomplicated measles.
- Ampicillin or other broad-spectrum antibiotic for secondary otitis media or pneumonia.
- Symptomatic treatment for encephalitis. Corticosteroid therapy may reduce cerebral oedema but of little value otherwise.

Prevention

Immediate
- Isolation: respiratory precautions justified in hospital until rash reaches staining stage; usually about 4 days from initial appearance. Not practicable elsewhere.
- Report to health authority; notifiable in UK.
- Contacts: household and other close contacts: live measles vaccine 0.5 ml i.m., preferably within 72 hours of exposure; normal human immunoglobulin (<1 year — 250 mg, 1–2 years — 500 mg, 3+ years — 750 mg) within 6 days of exposure to protect contacts at special risk, such as debilitated or immunocompromised children and those with cardiac or pulmonary disease. All school or nursery contacts should be offered vaccine unless they have a record of previous immunization.

Prevention

- Exclusion of recovered case from school or nursery until 7 days after onset of rash. Exclusion of contacts unnecessary.

Longterm
- Routine immunization (p. 357).

Meningitis

1 Aseptic

Organisms

Aseptic meningitis is commonly viral, but is also caused by myco-bacteria (*M. tuberculosis, M. bovis*), and, rarely by leptospires and fungi (*Cryptococcus neoformans* and *Candida albicans*).

Organism/disease	Epidemiology	Prevention
Enteroviruses (see p. 77)	Worldwide infections of man, usually symptomless in children, maximum incidence in summer and autumn in temperate zones. Spread by faecal–oral route. Commonest causal agents of aseptic meningitis	Poliomyelitis, routine immunization in childhood. Hygiene to prevent faecal–oral spread
HIV (see p. 133)	Worldwide infection particularly affecting homosexual men, i.v. drug abusers and recipients of contaminated blood products. Aseptic meningitis may occur at time of seroconversion	Counselling and education of persons in high-risk groups. Self deferral of blood donors and screening of donations
Mumps (see p. 186)	Worldwide infection of man, often symptomless. Endemic with epidemics every 3–4 years. Maximum in winter and early spring. Spread by droplets or contact with saliva. May be principal cause of aseptic meningitis in epidemic periods	Routine immunization in childhood
Lymphocytic choriomeningitis (arenavirus) (RNA)	Uncommon zoonosis; virus excreted in urine of house mice, pet hamsters and laboratory rodents. Spread probably by inhalation of dust contaminated with infected urine	Rodent control. Hygiene of household pets. Virological screening in laboratory animal-breeding units

Organism/disease/epidemiology/prevention

Organism/disease	Epidemiology	Prevention
Herpes simplex (see p. 129)	Very common infection of man, maximum incidence in young children. Spread by contact with infected secretions. Aseptic meningitis is a rare manifestation of primary infection.	None
Leptospirosis (see p. 153)	A zoonosis affecting particularly male adults occupationally exposed to infected urine of rats, dogs and other animals. Infection, especially canicola fever, may present as aseptic meningitis	Protective clothing. Hygiene in affected industries. Rodent control
Lyme disease (see p. 160)	Probably worldwide, follows distribution of tick vectors *Ixodes ricinus* and *I. dammini*. Associated with infection in deer, dogs and other domestic animals. Aseptic meningitis may follow primary rash or occur without rash	Clothing to prevent tick bites in infested woodlands. Tick control on pets and domestic animals
Tuberculosis (see p. 189)	Worldwide infection, spread person to person by droplet nuclei, cattle to man by milk, declining in developed countries where meningitis now uncommon. In UK less than 100 notifications per year and about 30 deaths. May follow primary infection in children or occur as part of generalized spread of infection in adults, especially debilitated elderly person.	Control of bovine infection by elimination of disease in cattle, pasteurization of milk. Control of human disease by early detection and effective treatment of cases, general measures to reduce exposure and improve health, BCG vaccination of at-risk groups. Routine vaccination in childhood recommended in areas of high incidence

Organism/disease/epidemiology/prevention

Organism/disease	Epidemiology	Prevention
Fungi	Rare causes of meningitis; usually in immuno-compromised or patients with shunts. Primary cryptococcal meningitis may occur in previously healthy subjects; fungus widely distributed in soil and pigeon droppings, spread by inhalation	Cryptococcal infection — avoid inhalation of dust from pigeon droppings. Candida (see p. 23)

Pathogenesis

Organism reaches meninges by haematogenous spread from site of penetration (commonly respiratory or gastrointestinal tracts) or of primary infection. Presentation often less acute and less severe than pyogenic meningitis; meningoencephalitis not uncommon with virus infections.

Clinical features

The incubation period and nature of the illness vary according to the infecting agent. There may be a prodromal period with general symptoms before signs of meningitis appear.

Viral meningitis

Affects mainly children and young adults. Sudden onset with headache, fever, vomiting and stiffness of neck and back. Mentally alert or slightly drowsy. Rashes common in enterovirus infections. CSF clear or hazy with a predominance of lymphocytes, slightly raised protein and normal sugar levels. Course usually benign unless there is involvement of brain or spinal cord.

Leptospiral meningitis

Sudden onset with headache, myalgia, epigastric pain. Oliguria and albuminuria in 40%. Slight jaundice common. Meningeal signs. May be encephalitic element. Conjunctivitis, iritis, scleritis or uveitis (see p. 154).

Clinical features

Tuberculous meningitis
Always secondary to disease elsewhere
Onset: insidious. Apathy, irritability and anorexia. Headache,
vomiting, abdominal pain and constipation. Irregular fever.
Second week: increasing neck stiffness and drowsiness, cranial
nerve palsies, choroidal tubercles 50%, papilloedema inconstant.
Third week: deepening coma, severe focal brain damage and
death.
CSF: pleocytosis with mixture of lymphocytes and polymorphonuclear leucocytes, protein levels high and sugar low. May be miliary
shadowing on chest X-ray.

Cryptococcal meningitis
Onset: insidious with symptoms for weeks or months before recog-
nition.
Early symptoms: headache, giddiness, irritability, impaired memory.
Follows fluctuating course. Often afebrile or low-grade pyrexia.
Minimal neck stiffness. Papilloedema in 30%. Cranial nerve involve-
ment. Fits and focal signs late. High mortality.

Candida meningitis
Neck stiffness and impaired consciousness. Difficult to recognize in
newborn.

Laboratory diagnosis — CSF

Macroscopic appearance
Clear or slightly opalescent, rarely cloudy, usually colourless, occasionally pale yellow tinge.

Microscopy and chemistry
● Cell count raised (usually 100−500/mm^3). Predominantly mononuclear response except in some cases of tuberculous meningitis and
in very early virus infections.
● Protein moderately raised. High levels may be found in tuberculous meningitis.
● Glucose normal or slightly reduced in viral infections. May be
greatly reduced in tuberculous meningitis and candidiasis.

- Centrifuged deposit should be examined microscopically if clinical suspicion of tuberculosis, cryptoccosis or candidiasis. Mycobacteria likely to be very scanty; cryptococci can be confused with lymphocytes but their thick capsules are readily visible in india-ink preparations.

Culture
Virus cultures or cultures for mycobacteria and fungi should be set up as indicated by clinical presentation.

Laboratory diagnosis — other specimens

Viral infection
- Cultures of throat swabs and faeces for range of aetiological viruses; specimens from herpetic lesions if present.
- Acute and convalescent sera for mumps and herpes antibodies, and for subsequent study against any enterovirus isolated.

Leptospirosis
- Diagnosis usually dependent on antibody detection (see p. 155).

Tuberculosis
See p. 192.

Treatment
- Symptomatic with analgesics and antiemetics.
- Specific chemotherapy for tuberculosis (see p. 193).
- Cryptococcal meningitis — amphotericin B i.v. and flucytosine orally for minimum of 6 weeks.
- Candida meningitis — amphotericin B for at least 6 weeks. Flucytosine may be given in addition to amphotericin if strain is sensitive.

2 Septic

Organisms
Pyogenic meningitis is caused by a wide range of organisms: commonest are *Neisseria meningitidis, Haemophilus influenzae, Strep-*

Organisms

tococcus pneumoniae. Enterobacteria (principally *E. coli*), group B streptococci, *Staphylococcus aureus* and *Listeria monocytogenes* are found more commonly in neonates than other age groups. *Staph. epidermidis* is particularly associated with pressure-relieving valves in hydrocephalus; anaerobes are rarely isolated. Uncommon organisms include amoebae (*Naegleria* and *Hartmanella* spp.).

Organism	Epidemiology	Prevention
N. meningitidis (see p. 182)	Worldwide endemic infection of man; periodic epidemics; affects mainly children and young adults; nasopharyngeal carriage common. Most frequent cause of septic meningitis in UK	Prevention of overcrowding in closed communities. Chemoprophylaxis of close contacts of cases. Immunization (groups A and C)
H. influenzae type b (see p. 112)	Worldwide, endemic infection, affects mainly young children aged 3 years or less. Nasopharyngeal carrier rate of 2–5%. Commonest cause of septic meningitis in North America	Routine immunization of children at age 18 months in USA. Chemoprophylaxis of child close contacts has been suggested
Strep. pneumoniae (see p. 289)	Common organism of respiratory tract of man. Meningitis may follow trauma. Affects all age groups	Chemoprophylaxis suggested in persons with recurrent pneumococcal meningitis (see p. 344)
L. monocytogenes (see p. 157)	Organism widespread in animals and environment. Worldwide uncommon infection; incidence increasing. Occasionally foodborne. Mother-to-fetus spread.	Care in animal husbandry. Pasteurization of milk and dairy products
Gram-negative organisms (see p. 43)	Commonest in infants and elderly. May result from hospital infection	Relevant to particular organism. Measures to prevent hospital infection

Pathogenesis
Bacteria usually originate from the upper respiratory tract and may spread directly, or via the bloodstream, to the meninges. They may also be derived from a primary focus of infection elsewhere by bloodstream invasion. Presentation depends on degree of infection, the inflammatory response and resultant increase in intracranial pressure.

Clinical features
Disease usually presents with sudden onset of fever and vomiting accompanied by neck stiffness and drowsiness but may develop insidiously. CSF rapidly becomes purulent. Mortality from bacterial meningitis remains alarmingly high despite availability of effective antibiotics. Features vary with age and infecting organism.

Neonatal meningitis
Vagueness of clinical condition renders diagnosis extremely difficult. Fever in 50%; meningeal signs often absent. Failure to feed and thrive; lethargy; poor general condition; respiratory distress; diarrhoea; jaundice. Essential to perform lumbar puncture.

Laboratory diagnosis — CSF
Should be collected into at least two sterile containers; the specimen with minimum contamination by blood should be used for microscopy.

Macroscopic appearance
Commonly cloudy or opalescent; rarely clear except in very early infection.

Microscopy and chemistry
Cell count raised (up to 4000/mm^3); polymorphonuclear response; protein increase in proportion to cells; glucose reduced or absent. Preliminary bacteriological diagnosis may be possible from Gram-stained film of centrifuged deposit.

Culture
Must include appropriate media and incubation conditions for likely

pathogens; anaerobic cultures included especially if meningitis secondary to abscess elsewhere or following skull trauma. All isolates are identified and sensitivities determined.

Laboratory diagnosis — other tests
- Countercurrent immunoelectrophoresis may allow rapid recognition of infection with meningococci, haemophilus or pneumococci.
- Estimation of CSF lactic acid concentration sometimes useful in differentiation of viral (<25 mg/dl) and bacterial (>30 mg/dl) infections.

Blood cultures
Should always be incubated from patients with meningitis.

Other specimens
Should be examined if clinically indicated (e.g. throat swab, sputum).

Treatment
- Depends on infecting organism.
- When no organism can be detected, chloramphenicol or ampicillin should be considered.
- Neonatal meningitis is difficult to treat because of the high resistance of many Gram-negative organisms and the toxicity of the drugs to the newborn. Appropriate antibiotics include ampicillin, chloramphenicol, co-trimoxazole and gentamicin.

Meningococcal infection

Organism
Neisseria meningitidis (groups A, B, C and others): fastidious Gram-negative diplococcus, closely related to *N. gonorrhoeae* (see p. 106). Human parasite.

Epidemiology

Distribution
Worldwide endemic infection; highest incidence in pre-school children, common in school children and young adults. Usually about 50% of cases under 5 years of age but proportion in older children and adults may arise during epidemics. Outbreaks may occur in schools and other closed or semi-closed communities of young persons, where susceptibles congregate. Community epidemics occur periodically, notably in sub-Saharan Africa where annual epidemics take place in spring, especially affecting the poorer classes.

Nasopharyngeal carriage common and duration varies with strain of *N. meningitidis*; overall prevalence usually 2−4% of population, may rise to 20% in epidemic times and to over 50% in outbreaks in closed communities. Factors which lead to development of disease not known but may be associated with secretory immunoglobulin (IgA) deficiency on mucosal cells, with passive smoking, or with intercurrent respiratory infections.

Group A strains common in Africa, northern India and Nepal; group A and C in Brazil; groups B and C in North America and Europe. Recent outbreaks of group A infection in Finland and Arabian peninsula, of group B type 15 infection in Norway, and rise of group B and C infections in UK. Over 1000 reported cases of meningococcal meningitis in UK in 1987 with over 100 deaths. Death rate highest in septicaemic cases without meningitis. In UK about 50% of strains are sulphonamide resistant.

Source
Human: nasopharyngeal secretions of cases and carriers.

Spread
Direct contact with respiratory secretions; droplets.

Pathogenesis

Majority of infections are subclinical and induce protective immunity. In some cases organism penetrates nasopharyngeal epithelium and enters bloodstream; spread to the meninges is presumably blood-borne. Infection frequently rapidly progressive and likely to induce disseminated intravascular coagulation (DIC). Later complications of arthritis and pericarditis due to immune-complex deposition.

Clinical features

Incubation period
Usually 1–3 days.

Acute septicaemia
Onset abrupt with shivering and rapid rise in temperature. Headache, nausea and vomiting, generalized aches and pains. Convulsions, especially in children. Rashes variable according to strain of organism: may be found in up to 50%. Fleeting macules or papules rapidly becoming haemorrhagic, or purpuric rash consisting of petechiae and ecchymoses. Some die; most (90%) progress rapidly to acute meningitis.

Acute meningitis
Violent headache, vomiting, neck stiffness and pain. Drowsiness and restlessness merge into coma and stupor. Non-epidemic meningitis less well defined and milder. Presenting symptoms very variable in young children. CSF purulent. Herpes simplex a common feature.

Chronic septicaemia
Recurrent bouts of fever accompanied by fleeting joint pains and crops of spots. Rash seldom profuse and consists of macules, papules, petechiae and even small vesicles or pustules. Either follows benign course, or occasionally terminates in acute meningitis.

Complications
Waterhouse–Friderichsen syndrome. Disseminated intravascular coagulation (DIC). Cranial nerve palsies, blindness and deafness.

Arthritis and pericarditis. Subdural effusions and hydrocephalus. Mental impairment.

Laboratory diagnosis

CSF (see p. 180)
- Polymorphonuclear leucocytosis, but if lumbar puncture performed very early in illness it may precede inflammatory response; culture nevertheless may be successful.
- Intracellular Gram-negative diplococci should be visible in stained film of centrifuged deposit.
- Culture deposit on chocolate blood agar, incubated in air with 10% CO_2.
- *N. meningitidis* identified biochemically or by immunofluorescence; subgroups identified serologically.

Blood cultures
Should be incubated without delay.

Throat swab
Cultured on chocolate or selective agar (see p. 108). Care must be taken to differentiate commensal neisseria.

Treatment
- Benzylpenicillin by intermittent i.v. infusion: 3 g 6-hourly.
- Chloramphenicol is a suitable alternative for patients hypersensitive to penicillin.
- Analgesics for headache; pethidine may be required.
- Diazepam or paraldehyde for the control of convulsions, followed by phenytoin.
- Fluid replacement.

Prevention

Immediate
- Isolation: respiratory precautions until 24 hours after start of chemotherapy.

Prevention

- Report to health authority. Meningitis and meningococcal septi-caemia without meningitis notifiable in UK.
- Surveillance of intimate contacts for 7 days after contact for evidence of disease and immediate chemotherapy if indicated.
- Prophylactic chemotherapy has been recommended for house-hold contacts (all age groups sharing living or sleeping accommo-dation with the case) and other intimate contacts, such as kissing contacts and persons in same sleeping accommodation in residential communities. Begin as soon as possible:

  Organism known to be *sulphonamide sensitive*: sulphadiazine (3 months – 1 year—250 mg, 1 – 12 years—500 mg, 12+ years—1 g) orally twice daily for 2 days.

  High level of *sulphonamide resistance*: rifampicin (3 months – 1 year—5 mg/kg, 1 – 12 years—10 mg/kg, 12+ years—600 mg) orally twice daily for 2 days. Ciprofloxacin 500 mg orally has been successfully used in young adults, when there was poor compliance with the 2-day rifampicin schedule.

- Prophylaxis is recommended for classroom contacts, if two or more cases occur in same class. The classroom contacts of a single case may have throat and nose swabs taken, and prophylaxis given if *N. meningitidis* of same group as the index case is isolated.
- Prophylaxis is not recommended in health-care staff unless they have given mouth-to-mouth respiration to an infected person, or have otherwise been intimately exposed.
- Immunization in outbreak (p. 360).
- Exclude household and other intimate contacts from work or school until 24 hours after beginning chemoprophylaxis.

Longterm
- Prevention of overcrowding in residential establishments.
- Personal hygiene to prevent spread of nasopharyngeal secretions.
- Immunization in epidemic areas and for travellers (p. 360).

Mumps

Organism

Mumps virus, paramyxovirus (RNA), related to viruses of Newcastle disease, rinderpest and distemper; causes cytopathogenic effects, lysis or multinucleate giant cell formation, in several tissue culture cell lines. Single serological type, but two antigens formed: V, associated with the virus particle, and the soluble S antigen.

Epidemiology

Distribution

Worldwide endemic disease; outbreaks in schools and recruit camps. Symptomless infection common, especially in young children; highest incidence in school-age children, in whom meningitis is an important manifestation, sometimes without parotitis; declining incidence in adults; rare in infancy because of maternal antibody. In UK, epidemics every 3–4 years with about 900 cases per 100 000 population in general practice; 100–500 new cases per 100 000 in non-epidemic years. Sharp decline in North America following introduction of routine immunization in 1970s.

Source

Human: saliva of case or symptomless excretor. Virus present in saliva for several days before and after onset of parotitis, and in saliva at similar period after infection in persons who do not develop symptoms.

Spread

Droplet or contact with saliva.

Pathogenesis

Virus replicates in mucosal cells followed by transient viraemia late in the incubation period before localizing in salivary glands, other glands or meninges. Causes non-suppurative inflammation.

Clinical features

Incubation period

Usually 18–21 days but may extend from 12–35 days.

Clinical features

Clinical syndromes
Many infections subclinical. Wide variety of clinical syndromes according to combination of organs involved. Severity and duration of illness very variable.

Salivary glands
Parotitis usually bilateral. Parotid papillae inflamed. Submaxillary salivary adenitis in 10%. Sublingual adenitis rare. Oedema of subcutaneous tissues produces jelly-like quivering.

Meningoencephalitis
Sole feature or associated with parotitis. Found in 0.5–10%. Usually benign but may be followed by permanent deafness in one or both ears (see pp. 69 and 174).

Orchitis
Usually associated with parotitis but may be sole manifestation. Found in 25% of men and adolescent boys. Unilateral in 80%. Sterility rare.

Other features
Pancreatitis 7%; oophoritis 5%; mastitis both sexes; prostatitis; myocarditis; arthritis; iritis.

Laboratory diagnosis
- Complement-fixing antibody to S antigen appears during acute stage, reaches peak during convalescence then declines; antibody to V antigen detectable somewhat later and persists longer.
- Virus can be isolated from saliva or throat washings during early days of illness; culture from CSF in meningitis also possible. Serology more useful.
- CSF: lymphocytic response in meningitis, sugar may be low.
- Serum amylase elevated in 70% of cases.

Treatment
Symptomatic. Corticosteroid therapy may relieve distress from severe orchitis but does not affect course of disease.

Prevention

Immediate
- Isolation: respiratory precautions until illness subsides.
- Report to health authority; notifiable in UK.
- Exclusion from work or school until clinical recovery.
- Contacts: no exclusion necessary. Immunization should be offered to previously unimmunized contacts. Normal human immunoglobulin is not effective in preventing mumps.

Longterm
- Routine immunization in infancy with measles/mumps/rubella vaccine (p. 358).

Mycobacterial infections

1 Tuberculosis

Organisms
The genus *Mycobacterium* includes pathogenic and non-pathogenic species: *M. tuberculosis* and *M. bovis*, equally pathogenic for man, cause tuberculosis and are aerobic, acid-fast (Ziehl–Nielsen's stain) rods. They require special media (e.g. Lowenstein–Jensen or pyruvate egg) and are slow-growing: species identification is based on biochemical reactions, pigmentation, growth rate and optimal growth temperature.

Epidemiology

Distribution
Worldwide endemic disease; localized outbreaks amongst susceptible persons exposed to infection in crowded enclosed spaces. Declining in many parts of the world, increase reported in some areas affected by HIV epidemic. Respiratory disease due to *M. tuberculosis* universal, but non-respiratory disease due to *M. bovis* rare in countries with tuberculosis-free cattle herds and pasteurization of milk. In UK about 5000 notifications and 1500 deaths per year 1980–87, declining by about 5% per year. Notification rates of respiratory tuberculosis in males twice that in females; highest in men aged 55 years and over and lowest in women of this age group and in children. Notification rates in Asian immigrants about 30 times that in white UK residents; about half this in UK-born citizens of Asian immigrant parents. Non-respiratory disease notification rates in Asians about 80 times that of whites; usually cervical glands, nearly always due to *M. tuberculosis*.

Source
Human: overt or subclinical case with bacteriologically positive sputum. In UK main source remains white males in age group 55 years and over. Tuberculous cattle.

Spread
Airborne by droplet nuclei. Indirect by dust rare. Direct implantation

into skin or mucous membranes rare. Consumption of contaminated milk or dairy products.

Pathogenesis
The form of disease depends on the immune state of host: primary and post-primary infections occur.

Primary infection
- Lesion develops at site of lodgement of organism (usually near periphery of middle or lower lobe of lung).
- Local polymorphonuclear and mononuclear response. Organisms are carried to regional lymph nodes (Ghon focus).
- Infection may extend via the lymphatics and thence the blood-stream to become widely disseminated (miliary infection).
- Ghon focus commonly heals, but may undergo caseation and progress to post-primary infection.
- Cell-mediated immunity stimulated, which modifies any subsequent infection.

Post-primary infection
May follow reactivation of healed primary focus, especially if im-munity wanes, or results from gradual extension of caseous Ghon focus, or from new infection. Differences from primary infection include:
- More chronic.
- Usually involves lung apex.
- Rarely affects regional nodes.
- If spread occurs it is by local extension, or via anatomical pathways (e.g. through bronchial tree), or via the bloodstream after erosion of a blood vessel.

Clinical features — primary tuberculosis

Infants and young children
Often symptomless. May be failure to thrive. Glandular component of primary complex predominates and bronchus readily occluded resulting in segmental or lobar collapse. Conversion from tuberculin negative to positive.

Mycobacterial infections: Tuberculosis

Clinical features—primary tuberculosis

Older children
Pyrexia and cough. Sensitization reactions, such as erythema nodosum or phlyctenular conjunctivitis.

Young adults
Lung component more marked than glandular. Pleural effusion now rare in UK.

Generalized infections
Discharge of infected material from caseating lesion into the circulation gives rise to generalized miliary tuberculosis and tuberculous meningitis (see p. 175). Usually follows within 6 months of primary infection. Once found most frequently below the age of 10 years, now more prevalent in young adults. Onset abrupt or gradual with severe general symptoms and high fever with disproportionate tachycardia. Tuberculous meningitis develops in approximately 90% of cases.

Clinical features — post-primary tuberculosis
Any organ may be affected though seldom the thyroid, pancreas, salivary glands, heart or skeletal muscles. For osteomyelitis see pp. 202—4.

Pulmonary tuberculosis
Very variable and the extent of the lung damage depends on the balance between exudation and healing: at one extreme a rapidly caseating pneumonia; at the other a chronic well-circumscribed cavity with much fibrosis. Pleural effusion and tuberculous empyema. Endobronchial tuberculosis with obstruction and bronchiectasis. Illness varies greatly and respiratory symptoms may be absent. Should be considered in any patient with persistent cough, haemoptysis, unexplained fever or pneumonia failing to respond to antibiotics.

Lymphadenitis
Mediastinal nodes commonly affected; bacilli carried along lymphatics to other regional nodes; fever and malaise may precede glandular enlargement.

Renal tuberculosis
Increased frequency of micturition, dysuria and haematuria; little constitutional disturbance.

Laboratory diagnosis — primary infection

Ghon focus
Laboratory confirmation rarely obtained.

Miliary infection
Vigorous attempts should be made to isolate organism (e.g. from gastric aspirate, urine, CSF, sputum).
- Liver biopsy sometimes valuable.
- Tuberculin reaction may remain negative.

Laboratory diagnosis — post-primary infection
Specimens
- Tubercle bacilli may be scanty; isolation attempts should not, when practicable, rely on single specimens.
- Specimens should also be cultured from other sites to exclude widespread infection (e.g. culture urine in pulmonary disease; culture sputum and urine in meningitis).
- Sputum should be obtained after early-morning deep cough.
- If sputum not obtainable, early-morning gastric aspirates or secretions obtained at bronchoscopy are alternatives.
- Urine should be early-morning complete specimens (i.e. not mid-stream).
- Biopsy specimens (e.g. lymph nodes) should be divided and the part for culture should be sent in sterile container without fixative.

Microscopy
- Negative microscopy does not exclude mycobacterial infection.
- Acid-fast organisms seen in clinical material are not necessarily tubercle bacilli.
- It is reasonable to make presumptive diagnosis of mycobacterial infection if seen in CSF, biopsy material or in sputum if radiological or clinical evidence of pulmonary disease.
- Non-pathogenic mycobacteria may contaminate urine or intestinal

specimens; microscopy for these specimens is not routine in many laboratories.

Culture
- Specimens with commensal flora are treated to kill non-acid-fast organisms, and to concentrate the specimen, before culture.
- Cultures are incubated and examined weekly for at least 8 weeks (longer from patients being treated).
- Positive cultures for tubercle bacilli unlikely before 3 weeks; some atypical mycobacteria and saprophytes may grow more quickly.
- Isolation of mycobacteria, if not obviously saprophytes, is reported to the clinician.
- Guinea pig inoculation now rarely used.

Identification and sensitivity testing
Special techniques necessary; in UK carried out at regional centres.

Treatment — pulmonary tuberculosis
- Culture and determine sensitivities of organism
- Initial treatment: triple therapy using rifampicin and isoniazid in combination with ethambutol or streptomycin until sensitivities of organism are known or for a minimum of 8 weeks.
- Continued treatment: isoniazid combined with rifampicin, ethambutol or streptomycin to complete 9-month course.
- Second-line drugs: capreomycin, cycloserine, ethionamide, prothionamide, pyrazinamide and sodium aminosalicylate.
- Isoniazid: a supplement of pyridoxine 10 mg daily should be given, especially to children.

Treatment — non-pulmonary tuberculosis
As above but continue treatment for 12 months.

Prevention

Immediate
- Isolation: respiratory precautions for sputum smear-positive cases for 2+ weeks after start of effective chemotherapy as judged by

clinical improvement; wound precautions for discharging non-pulmonary disease.
- Report to health authority; notifiable in UK.
- Search for cases possibly exposed to same source of infection, especially in childhood tuberculosis.
- Trace contacts of sputum smear-positive cases possibly exposed during likely period of infectivity. These contacts would usually be defined as:

  Continuing contacts in household, workplace or elsewhere.
  Face-to-face contacts.
  Highly susceptible contacts, such as children under 16 years and immunocompromised persons, who occupied same enclosed space as index case, especially if case had watery sputum, frequent cough or poor personal hygiene.

- Trace contacts of sputum smear-negative cases possibly exposed during likely period of infectivity; should include only continuing contacts in household, etc. and highly susceptible persons who had face-to-face contact with the case.
- Screening and treatment of contacts:

Age of contact	Screening	Reading	Treatment
16 years or less	Mantoux test, PPD 10 TU *or* Heaf test (see below)	Mantoux: 16 mm or more induration, Heaf grade 3 or 4	Chemotherapy
		Mantoux 11−15 mm induration, Heaf grade 2	Investigation: chemotherapy if other evidence of tuberculosis
		Mantoux: 10 mm or less induration, Heaf grade 1	No treatment: repeat test in 2 months after last exposure
Over 16 years	Chest X-ray	Evidence of tuber-culosis	Chemotherapy
		Normal	No treatment

Prevention

- Tuberculin tests:

Mantoux	Heaf
PPD 10 i.u. per 0.1 ml*	(PPD 100 000 i.u. per 1.0 ml)
(1 : 1000 dilution)	

Reading

72 hours (may be read up to 96 hours). Measure horizontal transverse diameter of induration in mm using transparent plastic ruler or callipers	4–7 days (may be read 3–10 days) *Grade 0* = no reaction or six faint marks on skin *Grade 1* = at least four small indurated papules *Grade 2* = an indurated ring formed by confluent papules *Grade 3* = a solid induration 5–10 mm wide *Grade 4* = induration over 10 mm wide, usually surmounted by vesicle or ulcer

Interpretation

Mantoux 0–5 mm	*Heaf 0.* Negative
Mantoux 6–10 mm	*Heaf 1.* Weakly positive: non-specific sensitivity, past BCG, or atypical mycobacterial infection
Mantoux 11–15 mm	*Heaf 2.* Positive: past *M. tuberculosis* infection, BCG or atypical mycobacterial infection
Mantoux 16+ mm	*Heaf 3 and 4.* Strongly positive: current or past *M. tuberculosis* infection

* In testing patients in whom tuberculosis is suspected purified protein derivative (PPD) 1 i.u. per 0.1 ml (1 : 10 000 dilution) should be used.

- BCG vaccination is not indicated as an immediate control measure because it complicates the use of the tuberculin test as a diagnostic procedure and because its protective effect is not immediate. Previous BCG vaccination rarely causes a strongly positive reaction (Mantoux PPD 10 i.u. 16 mm or more induration; Heaf test grade 3 or 4).

Longterm
- Case finding and early effective chemotherapy.
- Vigorous contact tracing of sputum smear-positive cases, appropriate screening and treatment (see above).
- Tuberculin testing and, if indicated, BCG vaccination (p. 358).
- Eradication of tuberculosis from cattle; pasteurization of milk.
- Improve housing and nutrition.
- Advise against smoking.

2 Atypical mycobacteria

Organisms
Mycobacteria that differ from tubercle bacilli (*M. tuberculosis, M. bovis*) and which may be human pathogens. Atypical mycobacteria are of low virulence; recognition depends on biochemical reactions, optimal growth temperature (30–33°C for *M. ulcerans, M. marinum*), pigmentation when exposed to light (*M. kansasii*), resistance to range of antituberculous drugs. Identification best performed in reference laboratories.

Epidemiology

Distribution
Worldwide, common infections, usually symptomless. Infection may cause tuberculin conversion and lead to difficulties in interpretation of positive reactions in the diagnosis of tuberculosis. Skin ulceration occurs in workers in aquaria, and in swimmers (swimming pool granuloma). Disseminated atypical mycobacterial infection is a common manifestation of Aids.

Source
Not fully known. Animals and environment.

Spread
Not fully known. Direct contact of abrasions with contaminated water in skin ulcer. No evidence of person-to-person transmission of pulmonary disease.

Pathogenesis
May be isolated from symptomless patients; when recovered from symptomatic patients, possibility of underlying infection with *M. tuberculosis* or *M. bovis* should not be ignored; should be isolated repeatedly from sputum before a pathogenic role ascribed; causative role in lymphadenitis and indolent skin ulceration more certain.

Clinical features
● *M. kansasii* and *M. avium-intracellulare*: benign disease resembling tuberculosis of the lungs in elderly men. Cervical lymphadenitis especially in children.
● *M. marinum (balnei)* infection: mild ulceration of the skin.
● *M. ulcerans (buruli)* infection: slowly spreading indolent ulcers reported from country dwellers in Australia and East Africa.
● *M. fortuitum* infection: suppurative lesions.
● *M. scrofulaceum* infection: cervical lymphadenitis especially in children.
● *M. xenopi* infection: disease resembles pulmonary tuberculosis.

Laboratory diagnosis
As for tubercle bacilli; possibility of atypical infection should be considered for cultures unexpectedly negative after 8 weeks' incubation at 37°C; incubation should be continued at 30°C, especially if microscopy of original specimen is positive and organism is known not to have been exposed to chemotherapy. Cultures should be incubated at 37°C and 30°C from specimens thought likely to yield *M. ulcerans* or *M. marinum*. Sensitivity testing should be undertaken but it is not a reliable guide to clinical response.

Treatment
Response to chemotherapy unsatisfactory in 30% of cases. Continue treatment for 2 years. Surgery may be required.

Prevention

Immediate
● Isolation: respiratory precautions in pulmonary disease until

diagnosis has been established; isolation unnecessary in non-pulmonary disease.
- Report to health authority so that source of infection may be identified and controlled, particularly of swimming pool granuloma.

Longterm
- Good maintenance and cleaning of swimming pools.
- Care and protection of skin when working in aquaria.

3 Leprosy

Organism
Mycobacterium leprae: an acid/alcohol-fast, slender, very slow growing rod: culture in artificial media not yet possible, but growth in the mouse footpad and in the armadillo permit sensitivity testing: growth in tissue culture also reported. Low virulence.

Epidemiology

Distribution
Mainly in tropics and subtropics; estimated world prevalence about 12 million cases; common in India, South East Asia, Pacific islands, China and tropical Africa. In UK about 400 cases under surveillance; 10−20 new imported cases per year.

Source
Human. Nasal discharges of infectious patient.

Spread
Close and continuous household contact. No transmission in northern Europe.

Pathogenesis
- Intracellular parasite with predilection for peripheral nerve fibrils; characteristically found in dermis.
- Infiltration leads to depigmentation, disruption of hair follicles and sweat glands, disturbed function of peripheral nerves.

Mycobacterial infections: Leprosy

Pathogenesis

- Varied clinical manifestations largely due to efficiency and extent of cell-mediated immune response.

Lepromatous
Organisms numerous in skin, mucosa of respiratory tract and widely disseminated in other organs; minimal host reaction.

Tuberculoid
Scanty organisms; vigorous host response.

Borderline
Features of both lepromatous and tuberculoid forms.

Indeterminate
Early manifestation in skin, usually heals spontaneously, occasionally progresses to a determined form.

Clinical features
Incubation period may be 20 years or more.

Indeterminate
- Hypopigmented macular lesion (20–50 mm diameter) sited anywhere on body.
- No nerve damage.
- Heals spontaneously in 75% of cases. Remainder progress to tuberculoid or lepromatous.

Determinate
May arise from indeterminate stage or independently.

Contrasting clinical features of lepromatous, tuberculoid and borderline leprosy

Lepromatous	Tuberculoid	Borderline
Cell-mediated immunity weak	Cell-mediated immunity strong	Cell-mediated immunity unstable
Numerous ill-defined erythematous or hypopigmented macules	Few well-demarcated erythematous or hypopigmented macules	Mixed skin lesions

Mycobacterial infections: Leprosy

Contrasting clinical features

Lepromatous	Tuberculoid	Borderline
Later thickening of skin and formation of nodules	Diminished sensation in skin lesions	
Thickened nerves and peripheral anaesthesia	Thickened nerves with sensory and motor loss	Always marked nerve involvement
Nasal congestion and crusting	Trophic ulcers and corneal damage	Untreated cases evolve towards lepromatous type
Type 2 reaction: erythema nodosum leprosum, fever, joint and lymph node swelling, albuminuria and renal impairment, iritis and orchitis	Bone resorption	Treated cases evolve towards tuberculoid type

Laboratory diagnosis

Demonstration of organism
● Slit-skin technique: active edge of lesion incised as far as dermis; cells from exposed tissue expressed on to a slide and Ziehl−Neilsen stained.
● Scrapings from nasal mucosa examined similarly.
● Skin biopsy with serial sections may be necessary in tuberculoid infection.

Immunological
● Humoral antibody sometimes detectable using *M. lepraemurium*.
● Biological false-positive reaginic tests for syphilis in lepromatous leprosy.
● Lepromin reaction is of delayed hypersensitivity type but differs from the tuberculin reaction in that the main reaction develops after several weeks rather than 48 hours. It is strongly positive in patients with tuberculoid leprosy and is negative in those towards the lepromatous end of the spectrum. The test is rarely of value in diagnosis but useful prognostically.

Treatment

- Triple therapy for those towards the lepromatous end of the spectrum:
  Rifampicin 600 mg once a month under supervision.
  Dapsone 100 mg daily, self-administered.
  Clofazimine 300 mg once a month under supervision and 50 mg a day, self-administered.
Treatment should be continued for at least 2 years and ideally until smear-negative.
- Double therapy for those towards the tuberculoid end of the spectrum:
  Rifampicin 600 mg once a month under supervision.
  Dapsone 100 mg daily, self-administered.
Treatment should be continued for 6 months.
- Acute reactions: continue specific therapy and give prednisolone or thalidomide or aspirin to subdue reaction.
- Prevention of deformities: physiotherapy, relieve pressure on nerves, special shoes and reconstructive surgery.

Prevention

Immediate
- Isolation: wound precautions in lepromatous leprosy until infection is brought under control. Usually 2–3 weeks after start of treatment. Unnecessary in tuberculoid leprosy.
- Report to health authority; notifiable in UK.
- Investigation and surveillance of household contacts; early specific treatment when indicated.

Longterm
- Good housing conditions.
- BCG has been suggested for child household contacts but its efficacy varies.
- Chemoprophylaxis with dapsone 6–10 mg/kg bodyweight/week for 3 years has been recommended for child household contacts.

Osteomyelitis

Organisms

Acute infection
Wide range of bacteria but *Staph. aureus* responsible for 90%. Others include: *Strep. pyogenes*, especially in children less than 2 years old; *Haemophilus influenzae*; *Brucella* spp; *Staph. epidermidis*; *Salm. typhi*; *Salm. paratyphi*; other salmonellae, especially associated with sickle-cell disease; and anaerobes.

May occur also as part of generalized septicaemia, or by extension from infection in surrounding tissues, e.g. acute sinusitis. Osteomyelitis due to variety of organisms can follow compound fracture; mixed infections common.

Subacute infection
Mycobacterium tuberculosis, Actinomyces or fungi by local extension; occasionally atypical presentation of acute infection, especially after inadequate antibacterial treatment.

Epidemiology
See relevant sections under causative organisms as detailed above.

Pathogenesis
- Septic focus, usually in the skin, identifiable in about 10% of cases.
- Organism reaches bone via bloodstream; primary bacteraemia usually subclinical.
- Site of infection most commonly adjacent to metaphyses of long bones; configuration of capillaries possibly encourages lodgement.
- History of recent local trauma in approximately 40%; may have caused local hyperaemia.
- Secondary bacteraemia occurs.
- Untreated infection extends into marrow cavity and through cortex into periosteum, stripping the periosteum, eventually leading to involucrum formation and, through interruption of blood supply to cortex, to sequestra.
- Salmonella osteomyelitis in sickle-cell disease, possibly due to reactivation of residual focus of infection following capillary occlusion, e.g. in bone marrow.

Clinical features
- Haematogenous spread involves long bones of lower limbs or humerus in children and young adults; vertebral bodies in older adults; multiple bone involvement in small proportion of patients.
- Sudden onset in children with high fever and severe constitutional disturbance followed by signs of localized infection, especially pain.
- Adults may have similar onset or more insidious illness with minimal general disturbance and predominant focal signs.
- Older diabetic patients with vascular insufficiency may develop osteomyelitis of toe phalanges or tarsal bones.
- Mixed infection common in event of direct spread from wound, teeth or paranasal sinuses. Incidence greatest in older adults.
- Tuberculous osteomyelitis usually accompanied by arthritis of adjacent joint; chronic process with pain as presenting feature; spine a frequent site; ribs may be affected. Tuberculin hypersensitivity should always be demonstrable: positive responses are common in the general population but negative reactions virtually exclude the diagnosis.
- Radiological changes may not become apparent for 2–3 weeks.
- Technetium and gallium scans may facilitate diagnosis within the first few days and may demonstrate activity in chronic osteomyelitis.

Laboratory diagnosis

Culture
- *Specimens*: must be collected for identification and antibiotic sensitivity testing before treatment.
- *Blood cultures*: several sets should be taken within first few hours.
- *Site of primary infection*: nose and throat swabs, swabs from any skin sepsis. Tuberculosis: search for primary focus; examine sputum and early-morning urine specimens.
- *Bone site*: material removed at surgery should be cultured: needle biopsy of value in tuberculosis, both for histology and culture.

Serology
May be useful if culture is unsuccessful; see relevant sections for appropriate tests.

Treatment

Acute osteomyelitis
Commence treatment with i.v. penicillinase-resistant penicillin in combination with clindamycin or fucidin pending results of blood culture or needle biopsy. Adjust antibiotic regimen according to sensitivity tests and continue systemic therapy for minimum of 4 weeks.

Salmonella osteomyelitis
Amoxycillin or ampicillin.

Tuberculous osteomyelitis
Rifampicin, ethambutol and isoniazid for uncomplicated cases; surgery may be necessary for complications.

Chronic osteomyelitis
Prolonged treatment with appropriate antibiotics combined with surgical removal of necrotic or diseased tissues.

Prevention
See relevant sections.

Parvovirus B19 infections

Organism
Single-stranded DNA small viruses, approximately 20 nm in diameter. Parvovirus B19 recently identified as a human pathogen.

Epidemiology

Distribution
Probably worldwide; sporadic and in epidemics in spring; affects mainly children causing erythema infectiosum or fifth disease.

Source
Human.

Spread
Airborne: person to person, probably by droplets.

Pathogenesis
Virus enters via respiratory tract, viraemia follows and stimulates antibody response. Rash immunologically mediated. In bone marrow culture the virus inhibits development of erythrocyte precursors, presumably the basis of aplastic anaemia in sickle-cell disease (see below). Subclinical transient aplasia may occur commonly.

Clinical features
- Incubation period: 6–14 days.
- Prodromal period: short, may be absent. Mild fever, sore throat, slight gastrointestinal disturbance.
- Rash: appears first on face; blotchy erythema suggesting appearance of slapped cheeks.
- Secondary rash appears on trunk and limbs concurrently or within a few days. Appearance varies considerably from morbilliform to annular or confluent erythema. Tendency for rash to come and go over a week or longer; recurrence precipitated by hot baths, exercise or emotional upset.
- Usually benign illness in children but may be more severe in adults. Rash less prominent in adults and may be absent.
Lymphadenopathy and arthritis, especially of wrists and knees, are common in adult infection.

Clinical features

- May precipitate aplastic anaemia in patients with sickle-cell disease by damaging stem cells in bone marrow.
- May cause abortion or result in hydrops fetalis. Congenital defects not reported.

Laboratory diagnosis
- Serology: B19-specific IgM detectable during illness and early convalescence.
- Antigen determination: not routine; may be performed in laboratories undertaking parvovirus research.

Treatment
- Symptomatic.
- Blood transfusion for crisis in sickle-cell disease.

Prevention

Immediate
- Isolation usually impractical.
- Pregnant women and patients with sickle-cell disease should avoid contact with known cases.

Longterm
- None.

Pelvic inflammatory disease

A disease usually of young women due to ascending infection of the genital tract affecting the uterus, fallopian tubes and surrounding pelvic structures.

Epidemiology

Distribution

Worldwide, common disease. Usually consequence of post-abortum or post-partum infection with a variety of organisms (see p. 222) or of sexually transmitted disease. High incidence reported in parts of Africa. In western countries recent increase has followed rise in sexually transmitted disease and is probably due mainly to *Neisseria gonorrhoeae* and *Chlamydia trachomatis*; associated with increased sexual promiscuity and increased use of IUCD. Parallel increase in ectopic pregnancy. Chronic and relapsing pelvic inflammatory disease may be due to persistent symptomless gonococcal or chlamydial infection in male sexual partner.

In UK, hospital admissions for acute salpingitis and pelvic inflammatory disease more than doubled to nearly 20 000 per year 1965–85, and ectopic pregnancies increased by over one-third to over 4000 per year.

Source
Human.

Spread
Depends on organism. Sexual intercourse. Possibly endogenous. Indirectly by hands of attendants.

Prevention

Immediate
- Isolation unnecessary.
- Early bacteriological diagnosis and treatment.
- Gonococcal and chlamydial infection: identification, screening and treatment of sexual contacts.

Pelvic inflammatory disease

Prevention

Longterm
- Early detection and treatment of sexually transmitted disease.

Pertussis

Organism
Bordetella pertussis (three serotypes): Gram-negative coccobacillus with fastidious growth requirements; parasitic in human respiratory tract.

Epidemiology

Distribution
Worldwide, universal disease of childhood with highest mortality under 1 year of age, especially in poorly nourished children. May occur in adults, particularly in immunized communities. Incidence declined in many countries following routine immunization in infancy; rose in UK in 1970s following decline in immunization acceptance as a result of public controversy about vaccine-associated disease.

Source
Human: discharges from respiratory tract of children in the prodromal stage of the disease. School-aged children often the source of infection for younger siblings at home.

Spread
Direct contact with oropharyngeal discharges; airborne droplets.

Pathogenesis
Organism enters via the respiratory tract, adheres to epithelium of trachea and bronchi causing cell damage and interfering with ciliary action; does not invade bloodstream. Secretions and cell debris may block small air passages with resultant lobular collapse and secondary infection.

Clinical features

Incubation period
Usually 10–14 days.

Prodromal stage
Respiratory catarrh with simple cough.

Clinical features

Paroxysmal stage
Coughs become more grouped with series of expiratory grunts terminating in characteristic whoop or vomiting or both. Older children and adults may not whoop and very young children may have apnoeic attacks. Paroxysms in rapid succession may leave patient exhausted. Frequent vomiting may lead to progressive weakness from malnutrition. Temperature normal.

Course of illness
Very variable. Average attack advances for first 2 weeks, remains at a peak for 2 weeks, then abates over 2 weeks or longer.

Complications
- *Respiratory*: lobular or lobar collapse, bronchopneumonia.
- *Nervous system*: anoxic convulsions and encephalopathy.
- *Mechanical*: subconjunctival haemorrhage, fraenal ulcer, hernia or prolapse of rectum.

Laboratory diagnosis

Culture
Bordetella pertussis requires special media (Bordet–Gengou, or enriched charcoal blood agar); growth relatively slow, incubation continues for up to 4 days; penicillin added to prevent overgrowth of commensals. Identification by agglutination with antisera.
- *Acute infection*: pernasal swab the most satisfactory specimen; cough plates now rarely used. Specimens should be plated immediately on fresh medium; if impossible, transport medium must be used. Culture most successful in the incubation period and early in the illness.
- *Secondary infection*: sputum culture necessary if secondary infection supervenes.

Other methods
- Direct immunofluorescent examination of clinical specimens.
- Agglutinating and complement-fixing antibodies detectable from the second week of illness, but infrequently used diagnostically.

Laboratory diagnosis

- Blood count helpful in differential diagnosis; absolute lympho-cytosis a common and distinctive feature.

Treatment
- Skilled nursing to maintain clear airway and ensure adequate feeding.
- Mild sedation for frequent spasms.
- Oxygen for cyanosis.
- Antibiotics for secondary pneumonia.

Prevention

Immediate
- Isolation: respiratory precautions.
- Report to health authority; notifiable in UK.
- Exclude recovered cases from school for at least 3 weeks after onset of paroxysmal cough.
- Contacts: consider reinforcing dose of DT/Per/Vac/Ads for house-hold contacts under 7 years immunized in early childhood.
- School outbreaks: consider exclusion of unimmunized children with siblings under 1 year of age, whilst outbreak lasts, to avoid spread of infection to these household contacts.
- Hospital staff: exclusion from work if catarrhal symptoms develop.

Longterm
- Immunization in infancy with three doses of whole-cell combined DT/Per/Vac/Ads (p. 355). Acellular vaccines may cause fewer local and systemic reactions, although there is no substantial evidence that either vaccine causes permanent neurological damage; field trials of efficacy of acellular vaccines in progress; routine use in Japan at age 2 years supports their efficacy.
- Improved nutrition, general health, housing.

Pneumonia

1 Acute bacterial

Organisms
Acute bacterial pneumonia in the previously healthy is commonly caused by *Strep. pneumoniae* (see p. 289). *Staph. aureus* (see p. 271) and *Haemophilus influenzae* (see p. 112) are infrequently responsible, except post-operatively and in children and the elderly, but are commonly associated with viral pneumonia in all age groups. Aspiration pneumonia may additionally be caused by anaerobes and, following antibiotics, by enterobacteria (e.g. *E. coli, Klebsiella pneumoniae*) and *P. aeruginosa*; mixed aerobic and anaerobic infections also occur.

Epidemiology

Distribution
- Community-acquired acute bacterial pneumonia: a common worldwide disease which has declined in incidence in recent years. Frequently affects children, the elderly and persons with underlying disease; occurs as a complication of viral respiratory disease, especially influenza. Highest incidence in winter in temperate climates.
- Hospital-acquired pneumonia: common in the debilitated, immunocompromised and patients on chemotherapy.
- Aspiration pneumonia: frequently follows impaired consciousness; caused by inhalation of aerobic and anaerobic organisms of the normal flora of the upper respiratory tract.

Source
Human. Gram-negative organisms may persist in warm moist hospital environment.

Spread
Direct contact; inhalation of droplets; indirectly in hospitals by contaminated equipment.

Clinical features
The clinical symptoms and signs are very variable and may be considerably modified by previous chemotherapy.
    Community-acquired infections are usually caused by *Strep.*

Clinical features

pneumoniae or _Staph. aureus_ and less frequently by _H. influenzae_.
Pneumonia associated with aspiration may be due to less virulent
serotypes of _Strep. pneumoniae_, Gram-negative or anaerobic
bacteria.

Predisposing factors include chronic obstructive airway disease,
cardiovascular disease, diabetes, alcoholism and preceding virus
infections. Influenza is a common predisposing cause of staphylococcal and pneumococcal pneumonia in previously healthy young
adults.

Complications
Pleural effusion and empyema. Pneumothorax or pyopneumothorax,
especially in staphylococcal infections of infants. Bacteraemia leading
to metastatic infection. Meningitis important complication in pneumococcal pneumonia. Pericarditis. Renal failure.

Clinical features — acute bacterial and primary atypical pneumonia

Main features	Acute bacterial	Primary atypical
Onset	Abrupt or insidious	Insidious
Upper respiratory symptoms	Absent or trivial	Prominent
Sputum	Purulent, often bloodstained	Scanty, mucoid or mucopurulent
Physical signs	Prominent; evidence of consolidation	Minimal
Radiological appearances	Segmental or lobar consolidation	Prominent; segmental or lobar consolidation; ground-glass hilar flare
Pleuritic pain	Present in 70%	Uncommon
WBC	Commonly polymorphonuclear leucocytosis; may be normal	Normal or slight polymorphonuclear leucocytosis
ESR	Moderately increased	May be greatly increased>80 mm in 1 hour

Clinical features — pneumococcal pneumonia
Primary pneumonia now rare in Britain. Affects mainly age group 10–40 years and has abrupt onset. Continuous fever terminating by crisis. Pneumococcal pneumonia in children always lobular. Pneumonia due to higher-numbered serotypes found in extremes of life and in patients with impaired resistance (see p. 289). Endogenous infection from nasopharynx. Sputum viscous, purulent and blood-stained. Blood culture positive in 25%.

Clinical features — staphylococcal pneumonia
May be secondary to viral respiratory tract infection or to septicaemia. Always serious and may be fulminating. Ring shadows may be found on X-ray examination.

Clinical features — *H. influenzae* pneumonia
Found in older patients and in those with obstructive airway disease. No distinctive features.

Clinical features — klebsiella pneumonia
Most frequent between the ages of 40 and 60 years. Accounts for less than 1% of bacterial pneumonias. Tends to attack debilitated patients. High fatality and severe residual lung damage. Ring shadows on X-ray examination.

Laboratory diagnosis

Sputum specimens
Organisms causing pneumonia are commensals in the upper respiratory tract and therefore contaminate expectorated sputum; laboratory methods to dilute out contaminants are commonly employed. When possible, bronchoscopy or transtracheal aspiration specimens are preferable, and are essential for anaerobic culture. Sputum must be fresh, and expectorated after deep cough or physiotherapy.

Assessment of culture
• *Gram film*: prepared from an adequate specimen will show pus cells, very scanty epithelial cells and the pathogen alone or predominant; pneumococcal pneumonia recognizable in the Gram film.

Laboratory diagnosis

- *Culture significance*: determined in context of sputum macroscopic appearance, the direct Gram film, the purity and heaviness of bacterial growth and the patient's clinical condition. The antibiotic sensitivity of pathogens should be ascertained.

Other methods
- Examination of sputum for pneumococcal antigen by countercurrent immunoelectrophoresis may be successful when culture has failed; rapid test.
- Blood cultures from young children, the elderly and the very ill.

Treatment
See p. 221.

Prevention

Immediate
- Isolation: respiratory precautions depending on nature of infecting organism. Usually unnecessary for aspiration-type pneumonia.
- In hospital-acquired pneumonia, inform control-of-infection officer to enable investigation of source and spread.
- Report clusters of community-acquired pneumonia to health authority for epidemiological inquiry.

Longterm
- Improve general health and avoid overcrowding.
- Immunization with pneumococcal vaccine (p. 363).
- Influenza immunization (p. 363).

2 Primary atypical

Organisms
Clinical syndrome caused mainly by *Mycoplasma pneumoniae*; less commonly by viruses (see p. 217), occasionally by *Legionella pneumophila* (see p. 149); and uncommonly by *Coxiella burnetii* (Q fever) and *Chlamydia psittaci* (ornithosis) (see pp. 229 and 32).

Pneumonia: Primary atypical

Organisms

Mycoplasma pneumoniae

Mycoplasmas are cell wall-deficient organisms (therefore resistant to antibiotics acting on the cell wall), requiring enriched culture media and special methods for microscopy. Culture of *M. pneumoniae* is not practicable in routine diagnostic laboratories.

Human mycoplasmas also include two genital tract species of doubtful pathogenicity, *M. hominis* and *Ureaplasma urealyticum*.

Epidemiology — mycoplasmal pneumonia

Distribution

Worldwide endemic infection, occasional outbreaks especially in closed communities. Incidence usually highest in winter months in temperate climates. All age groups affected, but commonest in children and young adults aged 5–24 years. In UK up to 1000 laboratory-diagnosed infections annually, with regular epidemics every 3–4 years.

Source

Human, respiratory discharges of infected persons.

Spread

Direct contact with infected secretions. Inhalation of droplets.

Pathogenesis — mycoplasmal pneumonia

Not well understood but pneumonitis may be due to organism attaching to epithelial tissue and causing local necrosis.

Clinical features — mycoplasmal pneumonia

- Onset insidious with malaise, headache, shivering and sweating, myalgia and arthralgia.
- Upper respiratory symptoms followed by hacking cough with thick, mucoid sputum. Retrosternal discomfort but seldom pleuritic pain.
- Persistent fever but little respiratory distress. Few signs in chest. Occasional rash. Radiographic changes more striking than physical signs but not diagnostic: homogeneous ground-glass shadows, lobular and lobar consolidation. Sputum may become mucopurulent.

Clinical features—mycoplasmal pneumonia

WBC normal or slight polymorphonuclear leucocytosis in 20%. ESR>80 mm in 1 hour in 40%. Cold agglutinins in 50%.

Course
Fever gradually subsides after 7−10 days. Convalescence slow.

Complications
Haemolytic anaemia; encephalitis, myelitis and polyneuritis; myo-carditis; arthritis.

Laboratory diagnosis
Atypical pneumonia is confirmed by detecting humoral antibodies, preferably in rising titre, against one of the responsible agents. In 50% of patients with mycoplasmal pneumonia heterophile antibodies (anti-I) may be demonstrated by cold agglutination of washed human group O erythrocytes.

Treatment
See p. 221.

Prevention

Immediate
- Isolation: respiratory precautions until acute illness subsides.
- Report outbreaks to health authority to enable epidemiological investigation.

Longterm
Prevention of overcrowding in closed communities.

3 Viral

Organisms
Respiratory syncytial virus, parainfluenza and adenoviruses important in children. Influenza A and B important in adults, also adenoviruses 3, 4 and 7 in military recruits. Viral pneumonia may be a component of such diseases as measles or chickenpox.

Epidemiology

Distribution
Worldwide, endemic with seasonal epidemics usually in winter months but varies with agent.

Commonest in children, in whom it is an important cause of mortality and morbidity. Influenza is the principal cause of viral pneumonia in adults (see p. 143).

Source
Human. Respiratory secretions from case or symptomless child. Adenoviruses and enteroviruses in faeces.

Spread
Direct contact with infected secretions. Inhalation of droplets.

Clinical features
● Very common in children under 5 years of age; less common in adults.
● Very variable according to nature of virus and age of patient.
● Frequently commences as upper respiratory tract infection, which spreads after a few days to lower respiratory tract with deterioration in general conditon and increasing respiratory distress.
● Exanthem not uncommon.
● Radiographic appearances may be characteristic, as in chickenpox, or indistinguishable from bacterial pneumonia, especially in infants.

Laboratory diagnosis
● Attempt to isolate virus in tissue culture from sputum, throat swab or faeces as appropriate.
● Confirmatory diagnosis is usually by demonstration of fourfold rise in titre of humoral antibodies.
● Immunofluorescence may allow rapid demonstration of respiratory syncytial virus in clinical material.
● Failure to recover a bacterial pathogen from sputum may point to diagnosis of atypical and viral pneumonias.

Treatment
See below.

Prevention

Immediate
- Isolation: respiratory precautions until acute illness subsides.
- Report outbreaks to health authority to enable epidemiological investigation.

Longterm
- Improve housing and health of child population.
- Prevention of overcrowding.
- Personal hygiene to prevent dispersal of infected respiratory secretions.

4 Protozoal

Organism
Pneumocystis carinii, a protozoan appearing in the lungs as a cyst, approximately 10 μm in diameter, containing up to eight nucleated bodies.

Epidemiology

Distribution
First reported in 1955 causing 'interstitial plasma-cell pneumonia' in children. Later reported in immunocompromised patients. Outbreaks in homosexuals in 1981 were first indication of HIV epidemic. Very common manifestation of Aids; affects over 50% of cases; common cause of death.

Source
Human and animal. Epidemiological importance of different sources not known. Possibly endogenous.

Epidemiology

Spread
Airborne.

Pathogenesis
Most infections are inapparent. Disease due to multiplication of organisms and infiltration of inflammatory cells leading to distension of alveoli and disturbance of pulmonary function.

Clinical features
- Incubation period: uncertain.
- Onset of illness may be gradual or abrupt and fever may not be present.
- Respiratory distress out of proportion to chest signs. Progressive dyspnoea. Persistent non-productive cough.
- Initial chest radiograph may be clear but usually shows interstitial lung shadowing.
- Blood gas analysis usually indicates notable hypoxia even if chest X-ray is clear.

Laboratory diagnosis
- Demonstration of parasite by alveolar lavage or lung biopsy.
- Serological tests available but not entirely reliable.

Treatment
- Co-trimoxazole 120 mg/kg/day for 14–21 days, by slow i.v. infusion for first week then orally. Careful monitoring of blood, especially platelet count. Folinic acid, 15 mg on alternate days, may be given to prevent cytopenia. After recovery from acute phase treatment with co-trimoxazole 480 mg 2–4 times a day or Fansidar (pyrimethamine-sulphadoxine) one tablet weekly may help to prevent recrudescence of infection.
- Pentamidine should be considered if there is a severe toxic reaction to co-trimoxazole or failure of response.
   Pentamidine isethionate: 4 mg/kg/day as a slow daily i.v. infusion for 14–21 days; *or* Pentamidine mesylate: 2.5 mg/kg/day as above. Pentamidine is toxic and may precipitate hypoglycaemia.

Prevention

Immediate
- Isolation: usually not necessary unless to protect immunodeficient contacts in hospital.
- Report cases of Aids (p. 138).

Longterm
- None.

5   Treatment of specific pneumonias

Chemotherapy
- Pneumococcal pneumonia: benzylpenicillin.
- Staphylococcal pneumonia: cloxacillin or other penicillinase-resistant penicillin.
- *H. influenzae* pneumonia: ampicillin or co-trimoxazole.
- Klebsiella pneumonia: gentamicin or cephalosporin.
- Unknown cause: cloxacillin in combination with gentamicin or cephalosporin for severe illness. Metronidazole should be added when aspiration suspected.
- Mycoplasmal pneumonia: erythromycin or tetracycline.
- Ornithosis: tetracycline.
- Q fever: tetracycline.
- Legionnaires disease: erythromycin.

Other treatment
Oxygen; assisted ventilation.

Post-abortum and post-partum sepsis

Organisms

Exogenous organisms (such as *Strep. pyogenes* and *Staph. aureus*) and endogenous organisms (such as *Escherichia coli*, other enterobacteria, group B streptococci, enterococci, microaerophilic and anaerobic streptococci, *Clostridium perfringens* and *Bacteroides* spp.) are associated with puerperal sepsis; mixed infections, both of aerobes and anaerobes or of several species of anaerobes, are common.

Epidemiology

Distribution

Worldwide infections, affecting primarily the endometrium but spreading locally in the pelvis and systemically depending on the condition of the patient and virulence of the organism. Infection with *Strep. pyogenes* was formerly common but other organisms are now more important. Ascending infection by potentially pathogenic organisms, which comprise the normal flora of the lower genital tract, may occur following premature rupture of the membranes. Prolonged or difficult labour necessitating repeated vaginal examination, and retained placenta or incomplete abortion predispose to infection. Damage of the pelvic tissues following instrumental abortion predisposes to infection, including gas gangrene.

Source

● *Strep. pyogenes*: nose or throat of attendant or patient herself.

● *Staph. aureus*: often neonate, patient's own nose or skin, nose or septic lesions of other hospital patients or staff.

● Other organisms: the flora of the lower genital and gastrointestinal tracts.

Spread

Endogenous. Indirect by hands of attendants. Occasionally airborne.

Pathogenesis

● *Strep. pyogenes* causes severe, life-threatening infection, rapidly spreading locally and in the bloodstream (see p. 277); other aerobic pathogens apparently less virulent than anaerobes.

Post-abortum and post-partum sepsis

- Predisposing factors for endogenous infection include premature membrane rupture, prolonged labour and post-partum haemorrhage.
- Infection may result in a localized endometritis, or may involve other pelvic organs and the peritoneum.
- Severe anaerobic infection frequently causes pelvic thrombophlebitis, with risk of metastatic infection in lungs and other organs.

Clinical features
Puerperal sepsis may follow termination of pregnancy at any stage. Division into post-abortum and post-partum may be arbitrarily made when the fetus becomes legally viable.
- Pyrexia and tachycardia.
- Tender and subinvoluted uterus.
- Alteration in lochia, which is offensive with bowel-derived organisms; absent or scanty and inoffensive with *Strep. pyogenes*.

Spread of infection
Pelvic peritonitis or septicaemia. Staphylococcal septicaemia usually presents insidiously with metastatic lesions in heart valves, lung, bone or joints. *E. coli* causes transient or intermittent septicaemia, particularly following abortion. *Cl. perfringens* septicaemia is associated with rapidly deepening jaundice and may result in haemoglobinuria leading to renal failure. Anaerobic streptococci and *Bacteroides* spp. are commonly found in post-abortum sepsis and seldom cause fulminating illness.
Enterococci may involve the heart valves and prove difficult to eradicate.

Laboratory diagnosis
Proper collection and transportation of specimens is vital to recover anaerobes; contamination with vaginal commensals must be avoided. Tissue or pus, placed immediately in an anaerobic transport container, is far preferable to cervical swabs. If swabs are used it is imperative to use transport medium and culture without delay. Blood cultures should be taken, always including an anaerobic medium.

Culture
- Culture for aerobes and anaerobes.

- Complete identification and antibiotic sensitivity of all species present may be time-consuming; preliminary information should be available in 24 hours.
- Direct microscopy of Gram-stained pus may allow a presumptive diagnosis, e.g. of clostridial infection.
- Gas–liquid chromatography of pus useful to indicate presence of anaerobes.

Treatment
- Antibiotics after collecting cervical swabs and blood for culture and determination of sensitivity of organism. Initial choice benzyl-penicillin, gentamicin and metronidazole.
- Evacuation of retained products of conception under general anaesthesia 48 hours after commencing chemotherapy.
- Uterine haemorrhage can usually be controlled by ergometrine i.m.; blood transfusion may be required.
- Paralytic ileus: gastric suction and i.v. fluid replacement.
- Renal failure: Bull–Börst regimen or dialysis.
- Anaemia: gradually falling or persistently low haemoglobin level is indication for 1 u of fresh blood. Iron preparation should be prescribed for hypochromic anaemia.
- Salpingectomy or surgical drainage of abscess may prove necessary.

Prevention

Immediate
- Isolation: wound precautions when indicated by nature of infection.
- Specific chemotherapy.
- *Strep. pyogenes* infections: nose and throat swabs of attendants and close contacts, and treatment if organism is isolated.

Longterm
- High standard of antenatal and obstetric care.
- Rooming-in of newborn and early discharge from hospital.
- Strict asepsis in case of spontaneous and therapeutic abortion.
- Prevention of illegal abortion.

Pyrexia of undetermined origin (PUO)

Temperature taken by mouth in a normal person at rest varies between 36 and 37.5°C. Pyrexia of undetermined origin (PUO) does not have a generally agreed definition but may be regarded as any persistent fever which has been subjected to routine investigation with negative results.

● Cause of pyrexia in most patients is immediately obvious.

● In many unexplained fevers the illness is mild and of short duration so that lack of precision in diagnosis is unimportant.

● When fever continues for more than 5 days without apparent cause detailed investigation is essential.

● Investigation should be started without delay if the patient is gravely ill.

Main causes of fever

Infection
Commonest cause of fever. May be generalized or localized. Increased risk with extensive surgical procedures and use of prostheses. Importance of opportunistic infections in patients with impaired immunity due to drugs or disease.

Neoplasia
Fever common in Hodgkin's disease, other lymphomata and leukaemia; difficult to ascertain whether it is related to infection. Fever may be due to necrosis and autolysis in rapidly growing tumours, such as hypernephroma and metastatic carcinoma of the liver, or to secondary bacterial infection as in carcinoma of the lung or colon.

Collagen disease
Fever may be presenting feature and diagnosis may be difficult before other signs appear.

Hypersensitivity reactions
Infectious agents, drugs and foreign protein.

Other common causes
Sarcoidosis, ulcerative colitis, Crohn's disease, myocardial and pul-

monary infarction, thrombophlebitis, haemorrhage, haemolysis and profound anaemia, cirrhosis of the liver and metabolic disturbances.

Clinical features

History
Particular attention should be paid to the following.
- Onset of illness: gradual or abrupt; presenting symptoms.
- Pattern of illness with detailed chronological record.
- Symptoms referable to any system or region.
- Previous episodes.
- Previous illness: sepsis, rheumatic fever, congenital heart disease, surgical or dental operations.
- Family history: predisposition to disease, tuberculosis or typhoid fever in other members of family.
- Occupation, hobbies and animal contacts.
- Overseas travel or contact with person recently arrived from abroad.

Examination
Careful and repeated examination of all systems with special attention to the following.
- Skin: rashes and haemorrhages.
- Nails: splinter haemorrhages.
- Finger pulps: tender nodules.
- Heart: murmurs especially when changing in character.
- Reticuloendothelial system: lymphadenopathy, splenomegaly and hepatomegaly.
- Temperature: type and pattern of pyrexia.

Basic investigations
- Hb, total and differential WBC, ESR.
- Thick and thin films for malarial parasites when indicated by exposure in endemic area.
- Blood cultures × 3, aerobic and anaerobic; enriched CO_2 atmosphere when brucellosis is suspected.
- Bacterological examination of urine, faeces and any discharges.
- Microscopic examination of urine.
- Chest X-ray.

Basic investigations

* Acute serum to establish baseline titre for subsequent serological tests.

Further investigations
* Detection of autoantibodies, antinuclear factor or rheumatoid factor in collagen disease.
* Post-abortum and post-partum pyrexia: cervical and high vaginal swabs.
* Tuberculosis: sputum, gastric aspirates and urine for direct microscopy and culture. Mantoux test.
* Sarcoidosis: Kveim test.
* Needle biopsy: liver, bone marrow or pleura.
* Surgical biopsy: lymph node.
* Radiology: lungs, gastrointestinal, urinary and biliary tracts.
* Ultrasonic scan: liver and gallbladder.
* CAT (CT) scan: abdominal cavity.
* Exploratory laparotomy: fever for at least 1 month and main symptoms referable to abdomen. Should be considered earlier in the event of serious deterioration in patient's condition.

Interpretation of investigations

White blood cell count (WBC)
The WBC is very useful for classifying the likely cause of a pyrexial illness but must be interpreted with caution.
* Polymorphonuclear leucocytosis: pyogenic infection, leptospirosis, amoebic abscess and acute rheumatic fever.
* Normal WBC: virus or rickettsial infection. Enteric fever, brucellosis, tuberculosis, subacute bacterial endocarditis and severe septicaemia.
* Neutropenia: disseminated lupus erythematosus, primary disease of bone marrow.
* Eosinophilia: polyarteritis nodosa, lymphoreticular neoplasia, carcinomatosis of liver, worm infestations.

Interpretation of ESR
* Moderately raised in most infections but may be normal.
* Greatly raised (more than 80 mm in 1 hour) in collagen diseases,

myelomatosis, mycoplasmal infections, psittacosis, legionnaires disease and liver abscess.

Serology
Fourfold rise in titre of antibody in IgG, or antibody in IgM fraction against specific agent indicates recent infection.

Management

Persistent low-grade fever with no clinical or laboratory evidence of serious disease
Increase physical activity. This may:
- Produce exacerbation and reveal underlying cause; *or*
- Leave the fever unaltered without deterioration in physical well-being, in which event the temperature findings can be safely ignored.

Considerable illness with physical deterioration and negative investigations
- Repeat investigations frequently.
- Consider trial of antituberculosis drugs, such as ethambutol and isoniazid. Review after 3 weeks.
- In severe or life-threatening illness, when bacterial infection is thought to be the most likely cause, give a course of broad-spectrum antibiotic. If there is no improvement after 5 days change antibiotic.
- Persistent illness when a collagen disease or hypersensitivity response is thought to be the probable cause — therapeutic trial of prednisolone 40 mg daily under close supervision.

Q fever

Organism

Coxiella burnetii: rickettsia-like organism, but more resistant to heat and drying; cultured in chick yolk sac. Two antigens demonstrable, phase I present in freshly isolated strains, phase II in strains repeatedly passaged in eggs.

Epidemiology

Distribution

Zoonosis endemic in many parts of the world. Usually reported in male adults occupationally exposed to infected animals or their products in farming, veterinary practice, and the meat and dairy industries. Often sporadic, but explosive localized outbreaks are a feature of the disease. In UK, reported cases increased in late 1970s from about 50 per year to 150–200 per year in mid-1980s.

Source

Cattle, sheep and goats with symptomless infection, particularly placenta and uterine discharges at parturition. Wild animals may be infected and ticks may transfer the infection to domestic animals but rarely to man.

Spread

Usually by airborne route; inhalation of dust contaminated by animal excreta, or by placentae and other products of conception; may be transmitted by contaminated straw: the organism may survive in dust and straw for long periods. Direct contact with infected animals. Possibly milkborne. Person-to-person spread rare, has been reported in hospitals. A particular hazard in laboratories handling the organism or infected tissues.

Pathogenesis

● Pneumonitis common. Mononuclear cells predominate in alveolar exudate but less obvious in sputum. Some alveolar necrosis in severe infections; bronchioles also affected.
● Microcolonies demonstrable in vegetations of endocarditis at operation or autopsy.

● Hepatitis rare; may be only or early manifestation of chronic disease.

Clinical features

Incubation period
Extends from 2 to 4 weeks, usually 18−21 days.

Onset
Sudden, with acute febrile illness; malaise and myalgia; chilliness; severe headache, retro-orbital pain, neck stiffness but normal CSF; occasional confusion.

Other symptoms
Minimal respiratory symptoms and signs. X-ray examination may show areas of consolidation, usually towards end of first week.

Course
Fever settles after 7−10 days. Recovery 2−3 weeks.

Endocarditis
May be 5−10 years delay between acute infection and appearance of endocarditis. One-third of patients have underlying heart disease: congenital defect, especially bicuspid aortic valve; rheumatic heart disease; valve prosthesis. Highest incidence in young and middle-aged adults. Mainly affects aortic and mitral valves especially when damaged by rheumatic disease. Features of subacute endocarditis with negative blood cultures.

Laboratory diagnosis

Serology
Antibodies detectable by complement-fixation, agglutination or in-direct fluorescent methods; formed against phase I antigen only in long-standing infection; against phase II antigen in both acute and chronic disease.

Q fever

Culture
Blood and sputum culture possible during acute disease, by inoculation of chick yolk sac, but procedure hazardous and serology the diagnostic method of choice. Blood culture unlikely to be successful in endocarditis.

Treatment
- Tetracycline for acute attack in dosage of 1 g followed by 0.5 g 6-hourly until temperature has been normal for 3 days.
- Longterm treatment of endocarditis with tetracycline 2 g daily.
- Surgical removal of infected valve and replacement with prosthesis.

Prevention

Immediate
- Isolation: unnecessary once diagnosis has been established.
- Report to health authority.
- Search for associated cases, which may have been exposed to same source of infection.
- Epidemiological investigation and control of source.

Longterm
- High standards of animal husbandry.
- Pasteurization of milk.
- Care in handling laboratory specimens.

Rabies

Organism

Rabies virus: bullet-shaped rhabdovirus (RNA), approximately 180 ×
75 nm; one serotype. Grows in several tissue culture cell lines and
chick chorioallantoic membrane producing intracytoplasmic inclusions. Capable of causing disease in unusually wide range of
animal species.

Epidemiology

Distribution

Zoonosis, present in most parts of the world; Australia, New Zealand,
UK, Ireland, most of Scandinavia and Iceland rabies-free in 1987.
Mainly affects carnivores (foxes in Europe) and bats (vampire bats
in South America) and is transmitted sporadically to domestic animals, usually dogs, cats and livestock. All mammals susceptible. In
India and Africa common in semidomesticated dogs. Infection in
insectivorous bats recently reported in Europe.

   Human disease rare in Europe, North America and Australasia. In
UK since eradication in dogs at end of the 19th century, there have
been 19 imported cases 1902−87, 13 infected in Indian subcontinent
where human disease is very common with estimated 10−20 000
deaths each year. Common in other parts of Asia and Africa.

Source

Saliva of rabid animals, usually domestic dogs or cats, which may
contain virus for several days before onset of illness.
Semidomesticated dogs are a frequent source in Africa and India.

Spread

Bite of rabid animals, rarely by lick or scratch. Inhalation reported in
caves inhabited by vampire bats, and in a laboratory. Several reports
of transmission by corneal transplant from donors who had died of
unsuspected rabies.

Pathogenesis

Virus travels along nerves from site of injury to CNS, forms intracytoplasmic inclusions (Negri bodies) in neurones, especially in the

hippocampus. Some evidence also for centrifugal spread, possibly the route by which salivary and lachrymal glands are infected.

Clinical features

Canine rabies
- Incubation: usually 2–8 weeks extending to 8 months.
- Initial illness: change in animal's behaviour.
- Furious rabies: animal restless, excited and aggressive then uncoordinated and finally paralysed.
- Dumb rabies: animal quiet; difficulty in chewing and swallowing; coma and death.
- Duration of illness: 3–7 days.

Human rabies
- Incubation: usually 3–12 weeks depending on site of bite. Shortest incubation with bites of face. May range from 10 days to 2 years.
- Initial illness: headache, malaise, sore throat, anorexia, nausea, myalgia and slight fever. Most have pain and tingling at site of bite.
- Stage of excitement: acute anxiety. Fever and tachycardia. Difficulty in swallowing and sensation of choking, giving rise to hydrophobia. Some develop convulsive spasms preceding death; others develop paralyses followed by coma and circulatory collapse.
- Paralytic rabies: a minority, especially with bat-induced rabies, commence with paralysis in the bitten limb which extends and terminates with respiratory failure after 2–3 weeks.

Laboratory diagnosis
- Virus demonstration by immunofluorescence of brain from biopsy or at autopsy, of skin biopsy or of corneal scrapings; demonstration of Negri bodies in brain tissue less sensitive.
- Virus isolation by intracerebral injection of mice with saliva, CSF or brain tissue; examine at intervals after injection by immunofluorescence of tissues and histologically.
- Serological methods of limited value in early diagnosis.

Treatment
- Heavy sedation and analgesics.

• Intensive care, including tracheostomy and intermittent positive pressure ventilation (IPPV). Outcome very discouraging; only three reported survivors.

Prevention

Immediate — human case
• Isolation: strict.
• Inform health authority; notifiable in UK.
• Inform hospital control-of-infection officer.
• Contacts: health-care staff in immediate contact with the patient and other persons exposed to saliva of the patient should be given post-exposure treatment.
• Investigate and control animal source.

Immediate — post-exposure treatment
Following exposure from bite, lick or scratch of a wild animal, or domestic animal possibly infected with rabies virus or its health not known (especially if an unprovoked attack), in any part of the world not known to be rabies-free:
• Immediate thorough flushing of the wound to eliminate rabies virus; use soap or detergent (e.g. cetrimide solution 0.1%) and water or water alone, for at least 5 minutes. Then apply 40–70% alcohol, or tincture or aqueous solution of iodine.
• Appropriate surgical treatment; postpone suturing of wound.
• Passive immunization: human rabies immunoglobulin (HRIG), one dose of 20 iu/kg bodyweight, half locally infiltrated round wound and half i.m. (see below).
• Active immunization: human diploid cell vaccine (HDCV) in use in many countries — six doses of 1 ml i.m. into deltoid (antibody response may be poor following gluteal injection) on days 0, 3, 7, 14, 30 and 90 (see below); intradermal administration is not recommended for post-exposure treatment.
• Trace animal and ensure observation. Cease immunization if animal well 15 days after bite, or brain examined and shown to be negative for rabies virus.
• Advice on prophylaxis, and supplies of HRIG and HDCV available in UK from: public health laboratories, PHLS Virus Reference Laboratory

Prevention

Type of exposure	Animal and condition at time of exposure	Prophylaxis for exposed person
Minor bites of covered areas of arms, legs and trunk; scratches and abrasions; licks of skin	Suspected rabies; wild carnivore; unprovoked attack by any animal	HDCV: • If animal healthy at 15 days after bite or lab tests negative for rabies virus, cease vaccination course • If rabies confirmed in animal, also give HRIG
	Confirmed rabies or animal not available for observation	HRIG and HDCV
Major bites; bites of face, head, neck or hands; licks of mucosa	Suspected or confirmed rabies or animal not available for observation	HRIG and HDCV: • If animal healthy at 15 days after bite or lab tests negative for rabies virus, cease vaccination course

(tel. 01−200 4400) and CDSC (tel. 01−200 6868) in England and Wales; CD(S)U (tel. 041−964 7120) in Scotland; and DHSS (tel. 0232−650111 ext 758) in Northern Ireland.

Longterm
• Control dog population. Vaccination of dogs.
• In rabies-free areas: vaccination and 6-month quarantine for imported animals.
• Pre-exposure vaccination for persons exposed to risk:
  Workers in quarantine premises, laboratory workers handling rabies virus, veterinarians and other staff who may come in contact with rabid animals.
  Health-care staff in rabies units or who may be involved in rabies patient care.
  Travellers to remote rabies-endemic areas where prophylaxis unlikely to be available.
HDCV 1.0 ml i.m. into deltoid muscle two doses at 4 weeks interval and reinforcing dose after 12 months and every 1−3 years thereafter

depending on risk of exposure. If the risk is small this may be re-placed by three doses HDCV 0.1 ml intradermally at the same three intervals.

• It is advisable to carry out a serological test after pre-exposure immunization to ensure adequate antibody response has taken place.

• Pre-exposure immunization does not reduce need for treatment if bitten: thorough wound cleansing and HDCV 1.0 ml i.m. at days 0 and 3.

Respiratory infection (acute)

Infections of the respiratory tract cause syndromes according to the principal site of the infection. Pneumonia is discussed on pp. 212—21. Below are presented the main syndromes and usual causative agents. Epidemiology and prevention are similar.

Epidemiology

Distribution
Acute respiratory disease is worldwide, very common, particularly in children, and follows a seasonal pattern in temperate climates. Mortality is often high in infants in poor and overcrowded living conditions.

Source
Human. Respiratory secretions of case or symptomless carrier, often children.

Spread
Direct contact with infected secretions. Droplets.

Prevention

Immediate
Report institutional outbreaks to health authority to enable epidemiological study.

Longterm
- Improve housing and reduce overcrowding.
- Improve standard of nutrition in children. Maintain breastfeeding of infants.
- Personal hygiene to prevent dispersal of respiratory secretions.
- Immunization. Influenza in persons at special risk (see p. 363).
- Adenovirus vaccines have been used in closed communities of young adults.

Upper respiratory syndromes

Common cold
Very common infection caused by rhinoviruses and other respiratory and some enteric viruses. Endemic with epidemics in winter and spring in temperate zones.

Stomatitis
Common condition in children caused by Herpes simplex virus (see p. 130) and in infants and susceptible adults by *Candida albicans* (see p. 21). Cancrum oris, rare severe stomatitis in malnourished, debilitated children living in poor hygienic conditions.

Sinusitis
Common bacterial complication of common cold and other acute upper respiratory infections. Usually caused by *Strep. pneumoniae* or *Haemophilus influenzae*.

Otitis media
Very common disease of children. Usually bacterial infection with *Strep. pneumoniae* or *H. influenzae* following acute upper respiratory virus infection.

Tonsillitis and pharyngitis
Very common disease of children. Often caused by *Strep. pyogenes* (see p. 279); other bacterial causes rare, diphtheria (see p. 57). Vincent's angina in debilitated adults with poor oral hygiene. Frequent manifestation of viral respiratory infection especially with adenoviruses and influenza viruses.

Adenoviruses: endemic infections of children, particularly types 1, 2, 5 and 6. Virus types 3, 4, 7, 14 and 21 cause epidemic acute respiratory disease in young adults in closed communities. Epidemic pharyngoconjunctival fever in children, usually type 3 or 7 and keratoconjunctivitis in adults, usually type 8, are specific syndromes associated with adenovirus infection. In UK about 2000 laboratory diagnosed adenovirus infections reported annually 1980–87. Coxsackie viruses can cause acute respiratory disease; herpangina is caused by Coxsackie A viruses (see p. 79).

Respiratory infection (acute)

Upper respiratory syndromes

Croup
Common disease of infants and young children, usually viral in aetiology, most frequently parainfluenza viruses especially type 1. The latter are very common respiratory pathogens of young children: they are mild or symptomless in older children. In UK type 3 causes epidemics every summer, types 1 and 2 show an irregular pattern with a peak in the winter, sometimes in alternate years; nearly 1000 laboratory confirmed infections reported annually 1980–87.

Epiglottitis
Disease usually of young children but sometimes seen in adults including the elderly, caused by *H. influenzae*; high fatality rate (p. 113).

Lower respiratory syndromes

Influenza and influenza-like illness
See p. 144. Syndrome also caused by adenoviruses particularly in outbreaks in closed communities, and occasionally Coxsackie A and ECHOviruses.

Acute bronchitis
Common disease in all age groups often caused by influenza and other respiratory viruses. Rhinoviruses and respiratory syncytial virus common causes in infants.

Bronchiolitis
Worldwide disease of infants usually caused by respiratory syncytial virus, less commonly by parainfluenza and influenza viruses.
   Respiratory syncytial virus: universal infection, most children infected by 5 years of age. In infants under 6 months of age it causes acute bronchiolitis and pneumonia, in older infants and young children it causes acute bronchitis and upper respiratory tract infection, but in older children infection is often symptomless. Regular epidemics in winter in UK; over 1500 laboratory diagnosed infections reported annually 1980–87. Bronchiolitis and other severe infections more common in poor, overcrowded urban areas than in rural districts, and in artificially fed infants.

Lower respiratory syndromes

Pneumonia
See pp. 212–21.

Rubella

Organism
Rubivirus: non-arthropod-borne togavirus (RNA), 50–75 nm diameter; grows in rabbit kidney and baby hamster kidney cell lines; haemagglutination with avian cells; one serotype.

Epidemiology

Distribution
Worldwide, mild often subclinical infection, common in young children but more often seen in older children and adults than other childhood exanthemata; about 20% unvaccinated urban children aged 15 years non-immune in UK, but may be higher in Asian immigrant communities. Infection declining in USA following routine immunization in childhood since 1969; in UK where selective immunization of girls aged 11–14 years was introduced in 1971, epidemics have continued every 3–4 years.

Importance of infection arises because of its teratogenic effect first observed in Australia in 1941. Defects occur in most infants following maternal infection in first 7 weeks of pregnancy and are often severe, but defects have not been recorded in confirmed infections occurring after 17th week of pregnancy. Despite a high uptake of immunization in girls in UK of nearly 90%, an average of 20 cases of congenital rubella reported each year and up to 200 abortions carried out for rubella infection in pregnancy.

Source
Human: case, virus in throat for about 7 days before onset of rash, and a few days afterwards; subclinical infection; in the case of congenital rubella, virus may be shed for long periods.

Spread
Direct contact with respiratory secretions. Airborne droplets.

Pathogenesis
From respiratory tract virus spreads via regional lymphatics into bloodstream; transplacental spread from maternal viraemia; teratogenicity probably due to relatively low virulence of virus. Immune response important in pathogenesis of rash and of arthralgia.

241

Clinical features — postnatal rubella

Incubation period
Usually 17–18 days; may exceed 21 days.

Prodromal illness
Absent or short and very mild.

Onset
Headache, sore throat, cervical lymphadenopathy. Enlargement of suboccipital and posterior auricular nodes suggestive of rubella but variable. Grittiness of eyes and suffusion of conjunctivae.

Rash
May be absent especially in young children. Appears on first or second day of illness and fades within 4 days. Evolves from above downwards; first day consists of pinkish macules or maculopapules. Second day becomes confluent on trunk. Fades after third day leaving neither staining nor desquamation.

Complications
Seldom severe; arthritis or arthralgia in women, encephalitis and polyneuritis, thrombocytopenic purpura.

Clinical features — congenital rubella
Consequences of rubella in pregnancy are varied and unpredictable, ranging from fetal death to birth of an infected but otherwise normal child. Risk is greatest in early pregnancy and timing is critical in determining the site of maximum damage.

Temporary damage
- Thrombocytopenic purpura: appears at or shortly after birth. Initial mortality rate 35%. Haematological defect resolves in survivors.
- Low birth weight and retarded physical development.
- Skeletal abnormalities revealed by routine X-ray examination.
- Liver damage: progressive jaundice; generally resolves.
- Haemolysis: any time during first 6 months.

Permanent damage
- Heart disease: patent ductus, stenosis of pulmonary valve or artery.
- Perceptive deafness: may be difficult to recognize; prolonged surveillance essential.
- Eye defects: cataracts, retinopathy, glaucoma, cloudy cornea.
- CNS: chronic meningoencephalitis, microcephaly and retarded mental development. Progressive brain damage after interval of several years.

Laboratory diagnosis

Culture
Rubella virus may be isolated from throat swabs during first few days of illness, but is not routinely attempted. It may be detected in blood, urine and other body fluids of infected infants for several months.

Serology
Many tests are available for estimating rubella antibody. Single radial haemolysis (SRH) is sensitive and is replacing haemagglutination inhibition (HAI) and complement-fixing (CF) methods in many laboratories; other tests include latex agglutination and immunosorbent assay. Confirmation of acute infection depends on demonstrating a rising titre or the presence of IgM antibody.
- *Contact in pregnancy*: serological tests are performed as soon as possible.
- *Congenital infection*: confirmation of infection by detection of:
  IgM antibody in cord blood; titre continues to rise for 2–3 months after birth.
  IgG antibody in rising titre in infants over 3 months of age.

Treatment
- Symptomatic.
- Arthritis: rest and acetylsalicylic acid.
- Congenital defects: accurate assessment followed by specialist treatment for cataracts, deafness and congenital heart disease.

Prevention

Immediate

- Isolation: respiratory precautions for patients in hospital; outside hospital prevent exposure of pregnant women.
- Report to health authority. Rubella notifiable in UK. Congenital rubella in UK — report to Congenital Rubella Surveillance Programme (tel. 01−405 9200 ext 135, or 0532−452419).
- Contacts: serological screening of women in first 4 months of pregnancy (see below). Attempt should be made to confirm diagnosis in index case by serological tests.

Serum	Time of serum	Antibody results	Action
First	Within 10 days after contact	Seropositive Seronegative	None: reassure Repeat after 4 weeks
	More than 10 days after contact	Seropositive IgG only Seropositive IgM Seronegative	None: reassure Consider termination Repeat after 4 weeks
Second	4 weeks after first serum	Seropositive IgM or rising titre IgG Seronegative	Consider termination None: immunization during puerperium

- Human normal immunoglobulin of doubtful value; does not invalidate serological screening tests.
- Exclude from work or school until 7 days after onset of rash.

Longterm

Routine immunization with live-attenuated rubella vaccine. In UK in 1970 recommended for girls aged 11−13 years; in 1988 recommended for all children at 15 months of age, combined with mumps and measles vaccine (p. 358).

- Immunization of seronegative women at family planning clinics, in puerperium, and groups at special risk, e.g. teachers, health-care staff.

Prevention

- Immunization recommended for health-care staff of both sexes whose work brings them into contact with pregnant women, e.g. in antenatal clinics.

Salmonella infections

1 Infections other than typhoid and paratyphoid fevers

Organisms
Members of the genus *Salmonella*; apart from *Salm. typhi* and *Salm. paratyphi*. Several hundred strains, characterized by somatic (O) and flagellar (H) antigens (Kauffman–White scheme). Subdivision into 38 groups based on analysis of O antigens; complete identification requires determination of both phase 1 and phase 2 H antigens, using a range of antisera not usually available in routine laboratories; species designation applied to fully characterized strains. Phage-typing also available for some strains. Animal parasites.

Epidemiology

Distribution
Worldwide zoonosis; sporadic cases and outbreaks; very common in countries with intensive rearing of food animals, mass production of food and mass catering. Commonest cause of bacterial food poisoning in UK and North America. Almost continuous increase in UK since late 1960s, most evident during 1980s especially due to *Salm. typhimurium* and *Salm. enteritidis*; nearly 20 000 laboratory-reported infections in 1987. Many sporadic cases, but common-source food-borne outbreaks frequent and often associated with restaurants, canteens, hospitals and institutions; less than ten hospital outbreaks of salmonellosis reported in 1987; most hospital outbreaks due to person-to-person spread and are not foodborne. Maximum incidence in late summer and autumn; about 10% of infections acquired abroad. Severe disease may occur in very young, the elderly and in persons with achlorhydria; about 1.5% of laboratory-reported infections have extra-intestinal manifestations, such as bacteraemia, meningitis, and bone or joint infection; about 50 registered deaths attributed to salmonellosis annually in UK.

Source
Gastrointestinal contents of food-producing animals and less commonly of domestic pets and wild animals. Particularly common in

poultry and bovine animals in the UK. Human excreta rarely a source of foodborne disease, but often a source in institutional outbreaks.

Spread
Foodborne: cross-contamination of cooked products by raw foods, usually meat, poultry or eggs (particularly unpasteurized bulk egg products), previously contaminated by intestinal contents of infected livestock, then storage with inadequate refrigeration or at room temperature before consumption. Undercooking of contaminated meats/meat products, poultry/poultry products, eggs/egg products. Raw milk and dairy products. Contamination of food by an infected food handler is unusual; only likely to happen when the individual has diarrhoea and faecally contaminated hands come into direct contact with food not subsequently cooked. In these circumstances a small inoculum of organisms can grow rapidly in such foods as gelatine or cream. Person-to-person spread without the intermedium of food may occur and is common in hospitals and institutions, particularly psychiatric, maternity and children's units and old peoples' homes.

Environmental contamination may lead to persisting outbreaks, e.g. contamination in poorly-maintained refrigerators and kitchen equipment, in dust and cleaning equipment such as mops and vacuum cleaners, and in ward sluices and toilet facilities.

Pathogenesis
Variation in clinical features and their severity suggests interplay of different mechanisms similar to those governing intestinal pathogenesis of *E. coli* (see p. 97). Contributing factors include differences in host susceptibility, intestinal function, especially acid production in the stomach, and the number of organisms ingested.

Clinical features

Incubation period
Usually 12–48 hours, may extend to 7 days or longer.

Gastroenteritis
Common presentation. Varies greatly in severity and duration. Mild vomiting, severe watery diarrhoea, colicky abdominal pain, gener-

alized abdominal tenderness in severe cases, blood in stools in about a third of patients; fever, headache, malaise and generalized aching. Duration varies from 1 or 2 days to 3 weeks or longer. Tends to be exceptionally severe in debilitated patients or in those with achlorhydria.

Typhoid-like illness
An illness similar to typhoid fever may be found with any serotype of salmonella (see p. 251).

Septicaemia
Transient bacteraemia is very common with salmonella gastroenteritis but septicaemic features may dominate in any type of salmonella infection, especially with *Salm. cholerae-suis*.

Local infection
Systemic invasion may result in metastatic infection in any organ. Meningitis and osteomyelitis are not uncommon but endocarditis is rare. Sickle-cell disease predisposes to osteomyelitis. Local suppuration of the bowel wall and of the mesenteric lymph nodes is particularly common with *Salm. brandenburg* infections.

Laboratory diagnosis

Culture
● Faeces: methods described for *Salm. typhi* (p. 253), usually successful during acute stage of disease and for a variable time during convalescence; rectal swabs less satisfactory.
● Blood: should be attempted before treatment, in patients with features of septicaemia.
● Food: suspect food if available should be submitted to laboratory.

Serology
Rarely practicable because of multiplicity of antigens, inconstancy of antibody production and relatively late appearance in illness often of short duration.

Treatment
● Water and electrolyte replacement by i.v. infusion when necessary.

Treatment

- Graduated feeding.
- Symptomatic treatment with diphenoxylate or codeine for diarrhoea; metoclopramide for nausea.
- Antibiotics for invasive salmonellosis or local suppuration; ampicillin, chloramphenicol or co-trimoxazole.

Prevention

Immediate
- Isolation: enteric precautions.
- Report to health authority; notifiable as 'food poisoning' in UK.
- Epidemiological investigation to detect and control common-source outbreaks; most likely to be successful in clusters of cases caused by rare serotypes or bacteriophage types.
- In hospital: inform control-of-infection officer; bacteriological screening of all cases of diarrhoea and their contacts (patients and staff considered to have been exposed to the same foodborne source of infection, or exposed to faeces or vomitus of infected persons, or served by the same ward sluice or toilet facilities); isolation with enteric precautions of all cases and excreters; exclusion of infected staff from work (see below). Meticulous handwashing, aseptic preparation of infant feeds and special diets. Search for and eliminate environmental reservoirs of organism. Close ward to admissions if outbreak not controlled.
- Cases: exclusion of recovered cases and symptomless excreters from work or school, until bacteriological clearance (three consecutive negative faeces specimens collected at not less than 24-hour intervals), is usually only necessary if they are food handlers whose work involves direct manual contact with food to be eaten without further cooking, or are health-care staff looking after highly susceptible patients, in whom an intestinal infection would have particularly serious consequences, or are persons with poor standards of personal hygiene. Exclusion of other persons, who are well, from work or school is seldom justified.
- Contacts: consider exclusion of above categories until bacteriological clearance; exclusion of other categories of contacts usually unnecessary, and bacteriological screening unjustified except for epidemiological purposes.

• Prolonged exclusion from school or work, because of persistent faecal excretion of salmonellae, is seldom necessary provided that stools are normal and well-formed, and standards of personal hygiene are high. Each person should be considered individually and allowed to return to school or work as soon as possible.

Longterm

• Control of animal salmonellosis: high standards of animal husbandry, especially measures to reduce cross-infection; salmonella-free animal feeds.

• Food factories and food-processing plants: continuous education of staff, meticulous attention to hygiene, frequent inspection, bacteriological monitoring of raw materials and products, provision of chlorinated water supply, separation of raw from cooked products, pasteurization of milk and egg products. Irradiation of poultry meat has been suggested.

• Mass catering: continuous education and supervision of staff, meticulous hygiene, separation of raw from cooked foods, adequate refrigeration, full thawing of frozen products, thorough cooking of all meat, poultry and eggs.

• Public education in the prevention of food poisoning.

• Hospitals: bacteriological screening of children admitted to hospital; isolation with enteric precautions until at least one negative stool; screening of mothers admitted to maternity units has been suggested but this is not usually practicable.

2 Typhoid and paratyphoid fevers (enteric fever)

Organisms
Salmonella typhi and *Salm. paratyphi* A, B and C: human parasites, man the only natural host of *Salm. typhi*. Differentiated from other salmonellae by identification of flagellar (H), somatic (O) and, in freshly isolated strains, virulence (Vi) antigens; *Salm. typhi* also differs in some biochemical tests. Vi-positive strains can usually be bacteriophage typed, identical strains being sensitive to a phage adapted to that strain. Other *Salmonella* spp. occasionally become invasive causing a typhoid-like illness.

Epidemiology

Distribution
Worldwide infection, but wide variations in incidence associated with differing standards of hygiene and sanitation. Bacteriophage types show distinct geographic pattern and can often provide a clue to the source of infection. Endemic typhoid and paratyphoid virtually eliminated from North West Europe, North America and Australasia but imported disease common. In UK 150−200 cases of typhoid fever reported per year 1980−87, over 90% infected abroad; about 50 cases of paratyphoid A fever, almost all infected abroad; up to 50 cases of paratyphoid B fever, about 80% of them infected abroad.

Source
Human: case or carrier, usually faeces but occasionally urine. Paratyphoid B infection has been described in cattle.

Spread
Typhoid commonly waterborne; may be transmitted by milk, shellfish or other food contaminated by sewage (e.g. canned meat contaminated by cooling in polluted water) or by a single carrier. Paratyphoid usually milk or foodborne; may be spread by contaminated bulk foodstuffs, such as desiccated coconut and egg products.

Pathogenesis
After ingestion, during incubation and early clinical periods, organisms penetrate the intestinal mucosa and reach the regional lymphatics. Bloodstream invasion follows; organisms localize in gallbladder and Peyer's patches of small intestine, erosion of which may lead to perforation or haemorrhage; kidneys affected in about 30% of cases and other organs less frequently. Vi antigen apparently protects organism against killing following phagocytosis; lipopolysaccharide endotoxin derived from cell wall contributes to pathogenesis.

Clinical features — typhoid fever

Incubation period
Usually 10−14 days; may extend from 5−23 days.

Clinical features—typhoid fever

First week
Onset insidious with malaise, aches and pains. Epistaxis common; dry cough in 20%. Lethargy, anorexia, flatulent dyspepsia, constipation. Stepladder rise in temperature with relative bradycardia.

Second week
Pyrexia has reached peak. Rose-spot rash seen in <50% of adults; delicate pink macules or flattened papules, 2−4 mm diameter, over chest and abdomen; these appear in crops over a period of 1−2 weeks and last for 3−4 days. Apathetic. Abdomen distended; diarrhoea in one-third, loose yellow stools. Spleen palpable in 40%.

Third week
Illness critical. Delirium. Fatal outcome: haemorrhage, perforation or coma and circulatory failure. Favourable outcome: temperature falls by lysis, mental state clears, appetite returns and abdominal symptoms subside.

Variants
- Mild or abortive: apyrexial or short fever.
- Treated: temperature falls by lysis over few days and illness terminated.
- Meningotyphoid: meningismus.
- Nephrotyphoid: oedema, proteinuria and urinary casts.
- Pneumotyphoid or pleurotyphoid: signs of consolidation or pleurisy.
- Haemorrhagic typhoid: bleeding into skin or mucous membranes.

Relapses
Rate varies from 5 to 15%. Usually after 7−10 days of normal temperature, occasionally after 3 weeks. Attack similar to original but tends to be milder and shorter.

Children
Less typical and generally milder. Rash less common. Fewer complications. Gastroenteritis or asymptomatic bacteraemia in infants.

Complications
- Intestinal haemorrhage: 2−8%, usually in third week.

Clinical features—typhoid fever

- Perforation: 3–4%, usually towards end of third week; rare over age of 40 years; accounts for 25% of deaths.
- Others: cholecystitis, myocarditis, osteomyelitis.

Clinical features — paratyphoid fever

Paratyphoid A
Similar to typhoid fever.

Paratyphoid B
Similar to typhoid fever. Shorter incubation period. More abrupt onset. Duration shorter and illness milder. Vomiting and diarrhoea more prominent. Rash more striking.

Paratyphoid C
More septicaemic manifestations such as arthritis and cholecystitis.

Laboratory diagnosis

Isolation of *Salm. typhi* or *Salm. paratyphi*, ideally from the bloodstream, is the only reliable confirmation of the diagnosis; serological tests are at best supplementary.

Cultures
Blood culture: usually positive during early stage of clinical illness before treatment; progressively less likely to succeed from the end of the second week; reasonable to collect three sets of blood cultures during first few hours of investigation.
Faeces:

- Positive cultures expected from second week of untreated illness; cultures in earlier stages may be negative.
- Several specimens should be submitted, bloodstained or mucoid fragments being selected.
- Specimens are cultured on selective media; biochemical and serological tests are performed on non-lactose-fermenting colonies; 48–72 hours usually necessary for complete identification.
- Phage typing carried out only in reference laboratories.

Urine: entire early-morning specimens preferable to mid-stream specimens; centrifuged deposit cultured on selective media.

Other specimens: culture of blood clot may be successful when routine blood cultures fail, presumably because serum inhibitory factors absent; bone marrow, duodenal fluid, or other specimens indicated by clinical presentation sometimes useful.

Serology (Widal test)

Demonstration of a rising titre of antibodies to H, O and Vi antigens during the illness is supportive evidence of enteric infection; results on a single specimen are rarely useful. Determination of titre of Vi agglutinins requires considerable experience; comparison with a standard serum must always be made. Factors to be considered in interpretation of serology include:

- The stage of the illness.
- The effect of antibiotic treatment.
- Previous immunization with TAB (H antibodies persist for years, O antibodies more transitory).
- Level of antibodies, from previous or related infection, in the general population and ethnic group.
- Possibility of an anamnestic response.
- Occasional deficiency in one or more antigens of infecting strain.

Treatment

- Determine sensitivity of organism.
- Chloramphenicol still most effective drug. Should be given for minimum of 14 days to reduce incidence of relapse. Adults: 2–3g daily; children: 50–100 mg/kg daily.
- Amoxycillin 1 g 6-hourly for 14 days or ampicillin in similar dosage. Co-trimoxazole — four tablets (each tablet trimethoprim 80 mg and sulphamethoxazole 400 mg) twice daily until temperature settles then two tablets twice daily for 7 days.
- Corticosteroid: prednisolone 5–10 mg 6-hourly for gravely ill cases. Full dosage for 3 days then reduce and stop after 7 days.
- Liberal low-residue diet.
- Haemorrhage: sedate with morphine, nothing by mouth for 24 hours, replace blood.
- Perforation: treat conservatively. Light sedation, gastric aspiration, i.v. infusion, chloramphenicol by i.m. injection and by gastric tube.

Treatment

Surgery for perforation in convalescent patient or perforation with obstruction.

Prevention

Immediate
- Isolation: enteric precautions.
- Report to health authority. Typhoid and paratyphoid fevers are notifiable in UK.
- Epidemiological investigation; detailed inquiry, particularly of persons infected with same bacteriophage type, especially if type is uncommon in the area.
- Cases: food handlers should be excluded from work until shown not to be chronic carriers (12 negative stools over 6 months normally recommended), unless their job can be changed so as to avoid direct handling of food; health-care staff should be excluded from caring for highly susceptible patients; persons with poor standards of hygiene should be excluded from work or school; children under 5 years should be excluded from nurseries and nursery schools until three negative specimens at not less than 48 hour intervals; adults in other occupations and school children with normal standards of personal hygiene should be allowed to return to work or school when clinically well. Each person should be considered individually according to the precise nature of their work.
- Contacts (persons probably exposed to the same source of infection or to the excreta of a case): surveillance for 21 days after last contact and investigation if symptoms occur; exclusion from school or work unnecessary if symptom free, unless a food handler, health-care staff working with highly susceptible patients, or standards of hygiene are low; each contact should be considered individually; bacteriological clearance — three negative stools at not less than 48 hour intervals.
- Immunization: contraindicated in outbreak control because if given in incubation period may precipitate clinical disease.

Longterm
- Early detection and treatment of cases and carriers,
- Surveillance and education of chronic carriers.
- Pre-employment bacteriological screening of certain food handlers

(particularly if their work will include direct contact with food to be eaten without further cooking) and of waterworks employees who have a past history suggestive of enteric fever or of gastrointestinal illness contracted in an area of high typhoid endemicity, or who have resided in such an area for long periods. Pre-employment screening of other staff is unnecessary in areas where typhoid incidence is low.

● Hygienic sewage disposal; pure water supplies; high standards of personal and food hygiene; pasteurization of milk and bulk egg products; heat treatment of desiccated coconut; care to prevent post-processing contamination of canned foods; hygienic production of shellfish.

● Immunization: residents in endemic areas, travellers and laboratory workers (p. 361).

Skin infections

1 Bacterial

Impetigo

Organisms
Strep. pyogenes (p. 277) and *Staph. aureus* (p. 271).

Epidemiology

Distribution
Usually due to *Strep. pyogenes*; worldwide, endemic, common infection in children especially those living in overcrowded unhygienic conditions and in warm climates; seasonal peak in late summer in temperate climates. Outbreaks reported in schools, in adult closed communities such as mental institutions, military camps and prisons, in meat handlers and among athletic teams ('scrumpox' in rugger players). Sometimes due to nephritogenic type M strains of *Strep. pyogenes*.

   Staph. aureus also may cause impetigo alone or as a mixed infection. In newborn and infants severe staphylococcal skin disease may occur — bullous impetigo and scalded-skin syndrome (p. 273).

Source
Human skin lesions or asymptomatic skin carriage.

Spread
Direct or indirect contact. Spreads very readily amongst young children and in institutions.

Pathogenesis
- *Staph. aureus*: see p. 272.
- *Strep. pyogenes*: see p. 278.

Clinical features
- May affect apparently normal skin or complicate some underlying skin condition, such as pediculosis, scabies or acute fungus infection.

Impetigo

- Commonly starts on the face around mouth or nose and may spread rapidly to other parts of the body.
- Thick golden-yellow crust with streptococcal impetigo.
- Bullae or pustules, later forming crusts in staphylococcal impetigo.

Laboratory diagnosis
Isolation of responsible species by culture of pus or swab sample from active lesions. Demonstration of specific toxins, such as exfoliatin (p. 271), not undertaken routinely.

Treatment
- Trivial streptococcal or staphylococcal infections: local applications of antiseptic creams.
- Widespread streptococcal infection: systemic benzyl- or phenoxymethyl penicillin.
- Severe staphylococcal or mixed infections: penicillinase-resistant penicillin systemically.
- Note importance of treating any underlying condition.

Prevention

Immediate
- Isolation: wound precautions.
- Early specific treatment.
- Exclusion from schools until at least 24 hours after beginning antibiotic treatment.

Longterm
- Early detection and treatment of cases.
- Hygiene in schools and institutions separate towels and flannels; high standard of cleanliness.

Erysipelas
An uncommon manifestation of streptococcal skin infection; usually affects adults in temperate zones in winter months (see p. 280).

Erysipeloid

Organism
Erysipelothrix rhusiopathiae: Gram-positive rod, morphologically resembling corynebacteria.

Epidemiology

Distribution
Uncommon occupational zoonosis affecting farm workers and persons handling meat and fish. Usually sporadic, rare outbreaks reported. In UK less than ten laboratory diagnosed cases reported 1978–87.

Source
Widespread infection in animals; causes swine erysipelas in pigs. Also found in soil.

Spread
Direct contact with abraded skin.

Pathogenesis
Infection ordinarily remains localized; occasionally lymphangitis and lymphadenitis develop; rarely infection becomes generalized, producing septicaemia.

Clinical features
- Incubation period: 1–4 days.
- Little or no fever or constitutional disturbance.
- Localized lesion, often at site of abrasion; small reddened slightly raised area; extends peripherally as it fades in centre. No suppuration. Swelling, itching and pain.
- Regional lymphangitis and adenitis.
- Arthritis in adjacent joints in 6% of cases.
- Rarely septicaemia or endocarditis.
- Reinfection common.

Laboratory diagnosis
Isolation of organism from culture of skin biopsy; in rare septicaemic cases isolated from blood culture.

Treatment
Benzylpenicillin.

Prevention

Immediate
- Isolation unnecessary.
- None.

Longterm
- Hygiene in meat and fish trades; protective clothing, frequent handwashing.

Pseudomonas aeruginosa dermatitis

Organism
Pseudomonas aeruginosa: flagellated, aerobic, Gram-negative rod; thrives in moist environment; grows on simple culture medium, producing a blue-green pigment.

Epidemiology

Distribution
'Swimming pool rash' affects swimmers in poorly maintained heated swimming pools and whirlpool spas. Follows maceration of skin after prolonged immersion.

Source
Probably human.

Spread
Contact with contaminated water. May be endogenous.

Pseudomonas aeruginosa dermatitis

Pathogenesis
Dermonecrotizing toxin produced by many strains of *Ps. aeruginosa* but its precise role in skin infections not yet determined.

Clinical features
• Maceration of skin with superimposed maculopapular or vesiculo-pustular rash; severe infection in the immunocompromised.
• Otitis externa (swimmer's ear). Malignant otitis externa with invasion of surrounding tissues in elderly diabetics.

Laboratory diagnosis
Isolation of organism by culture of appropriate clinical specimens.

Treatment
• Swimming pool rash: subsides without requiring antibiotic therapy. No swimming until skin heals. Keep skin dry.
• Otitis externa: insert a ribbon gauze soaked in an astringent, such as aluminium acetate solution (8%), and keep gauze moist; eardrops containing aminoglycosides or polymyxin B should be used with care especially if the eardrum is perforated.
• Malignant otitis externa: systemic antibiotics according to sensitivity of organism (carbenicillin, ticarcillin, azlocillin, or piperacillin with or without aminoglycoside).

Prevention

Immediate
• Isolation: unnecessary.
• Case searching to identify case clusters.
• Investigation and treatment of source pool.

Longterm
• Hygienic maintenance of swimming pools and whirlpool spas.

Swimming pool granuloma
Mycobacterial infection (see p. 196).

Anthrax
See p. 8.

Diphtheria
See p. 57.

2 Fungal

Organisms
Dermatophytes: filamentous fungi of the genera *Microsporum,
Trichophyton, Epidermophyton.*

Epidemiology

Distribution
Worldwide infections, particularly common in warm climates. Ringworm of scalp common in young children, among whom institutional
outbreaks occur. Tinea cruris common in adult males in warm weather
associated with poorly fitting clothing limiting circulation of air. Tinea
pedis (athlete's foot) very common in children and young adults,
associated with swimming pools.

Source
Trichophyton capitis — often animals (especially dogs, cats and
cattle). *T. cruris* and *T. pedis* — human infection.

Spread
Direct or indirect contact.

Pathogenesis
Fungal hyphae penetrate superficial keratinized tissues. Extent of
immune response varies with species of fungus: those engendering
less active response more likely to cause chronic infection; more
active may induce hypersensitivity 'id' reaction.

Clinical features

Tinea capitis — non-inflammatory
- Usually associated with human-derived fungi.
- Multiple bald patches.
- Scaliness and stubble of broken hairs.
- No general disturbance.

Tinea capitis — inflammatory
- Particularly common with animal-derived fungi.
- Erythema and scaliness of scalp.
- Varies in severity from mild folliculitis to suppurative lesion (kerion).
- Fever, general malaise and regional lymphadenitis in the severest cases.
- Hair usually regrows; occasionally permanent baldness.

Tinea corporis
- Red annular lesions spreading outwards.
- Edge consists of scales, vesicles or pustules.
- Centre of lesion normal appearance or scaly.
- Lesion itchy but no general upset.

Tinea cruris
- Occurs mainly in males.
- Similar to tinea corporis but involves the skin around the groin and inner aspect of thighs. Avoids penis and scrotum.

Tinea pedis
- Maceration of skin between outer toes; *or*
- Deep-seated vesicular eruption on soles; *or*
- Dry scaly lesions on soles.

Tinea unguum
- White discoloration of nail.
- Subungual hyperkeratosis with separation of nail plate from bed.
- Nail friable and thickened.

Clinical features

Tinea barbae
- Scaly red circinate lesions without hair loss; *or*
- Pustular folliculitis with loss of hair.

Candidiasis
See p. 21.

Laboratory diagnosis
Skin scrapings, nail clippings or hairs plucked from affected sites examined by microscopy and culture.
- Microscopy: potassium hydroxide slide preparation examined for branching hyphae and arthrospores.

Treatment
- Local applications of miconazole, clotrimazole or econazole; or compound benzoic acid (Whitfield's) ointment for tinea corporis, cruris and pedis.
- Griseofulvin for tinea capitis and barbae (for at least 6–8 weeks); tinea of finger nails (3–4 months) and toe nails (at least 6 months). Dosage: 0.5–1 g daily by mouth.

Prevention

Immediate
- Isolation: wound precautions in hospital for tinea capitis; otherwise unnecessary.
- Report tinea of scalp to health authority to enable investigation of the source and spread.
- In school outbreaks, screen children under Wood's ultraviolet light to detect infected children.
- Exclude infected children with *T. capitis* until adequately treated; unnecessary to exclude children with tinea corporis provided treatment is given and lesions are covered; exclusion of children with *T. pedis* unnecessary.

Longterm
- Avoid contact with infected animals.
- Individual hairbrushes and towels in schools.

Prevention

- Hygiene and maintenance of swimming pool surrounds, dressing rooms and shower rooms.
- Personal hygiene to prevent maceration of skin.

3 Viral

Organisms
Human papilloma viruses responsible for warts. Pox viruses responsible for molluscum contagiosum, cowpox, orf and vaccinial infections.

Epidemiology

Distribution
- *Herpes simplex*: see p. 129.
- *Warts*: different types of papilloma virus appear to be tissue specific. Plantar warts very common in children and young adults. Warts in other areas of skin common in children. Venereal warts common in young adults; may be associated with carcinoma of cervix; in UK clinic reports increased during 1970s and 1980s; over 60 000 cases in 1986; rise in death rate from carcinoma of cervix in young women seen 1950−86.
- *Molluscum contagiosum*: worldwide, common in children on trunk or face, and in young adults in pubic region.
- *Cowpox, paravaccinia, orf*: zoonoses; probably worldwide; usually acquired by farmers, shepherds, veterinarians and abattoir workers.
- *Vaccinia*: vaccination against smallpox or spread from vaccinee; severe generalized disease may occur in eczematous subjects (eczema vaccinatum); smallpox vaccination no longer necessary except in persons working with pox viruses.

Source
- *Herpes simplex*: see p. 129.
- *Warts*: human.
- *Molluscum contagiosum*: human.
- *Cowpox, paravaccinia, orf*: sheep, goats and cattle; cat may be primary host of cowpox.
- *Vaccinia*: human.

Spread
- *Herpes simplex*: see p. 129.
- *Warts*: plantar warts indirect contact through floors and duck-boards in swimming pools; venereal warts, direct contact, sexual transmission.
- *Molluscum contagiosum*: direct contact, fomites, sexual transmission.
- *Cowpox, paravaccinia, orf*: direct contact with abraded skin.
- *Vaccinia*: accidental inoculation, direct contact.

Pathogenesis
Human papilloma viruses infect keratocytes, which proliferate to form benign tumours.

Pox virus lesions due to virus replication in basal layers of the epithelium with 'ballooning' degeneration of the cytoplasm forming vacuoles. Breakdown of cell membranes leads to coalescence of vacuoles and formation of vesicles.

Clinical features

Herpes simplex
See p. 130.

Molluscum contagiosum
- Generalized in young children and affects genital area in adults.
- Round swelling resembling pearl which varies in size from pinhead to pea; shallow central umbilication; contains creamy mass.
- Secondary infection may be found in large lesions.
- No constitutional disturbance.

Cowpox
Discrete firm pinkish nodules progressing to vesiculation and pustulation. Fever and lymphadenopathy. Heals in 6–8 weeks.

Paravaccinia
Granuloma. No liquefaction. Associated with severe allergic rashes. Heals in 2–3 weeks.

Clinical features

Orf
Erythema and papule progressing slowly to flat haemorrhagic blister; usually painless; no constitutional disturbance. Heals in 3−4 weeks without scar.

Vaccinia
Local pustular lesion of skin or mucosae with tendency to spread, giving rise to satellite lesions. Primary lesion heals leaving foveated scar. Eczema vaccinatum. Generalized infection in immunocompromised. Abortion and congenital infection.

Laboratory diagnosis
Not usually undertaken. Vesicular fluid and scrapings from the base of lesions may be taken for examination. Virus particles demonstrable in infected cells by electron microscopy. Some of the viruses may be grown on tissue culture.

Treatment
- Herpes simplex: see p. 131.
- Warts: chemical cauterization, curettage, cryotherapy.
- Molluscum contagiosum: curettage; local application of 12% salicylic acid; cryotherapy.
- Pox infections: symptomatic; hyperimmune globulin and thiosemicarbazone for severe vaccinia infection.

Prevention

Immediate
- Herpes simplex: see p. 132.
- Warts: in epidemics of plantar warts in schools, exclusion of affected children from swimming and other barefoot activities rarely justified; socks recommended in gymnasiums.
- Molluscum contagiosum: none.
- Cowpox, orf, paravaccinia: none.
- Vaccinia: isolation usually unnecessary unless disease extensive, as in eczema vaccinatum. Individual lesion should be covered by protective dressing until crusted.

Prevention

Longterm
- Herpes simplex: see p. 132.
- Warts: hygiene and maintenance of swimming pool surrounds to prevent spread of plantar warts; education on sexual transmission of warts.
- Molluscum contagiosum: avoid contact with lesions.
- Cowpox, orf, paravaccinia: avoid contact with lesions of animals; hygiene and hand washing in occupationally exposed persons.
- Vaccinia: limit vaccination, avoid contact with lesions.

4 Parasitic

Organisms
Pediculosis: *Pediculus humanus capitis* and *corporis*; *Phthirus pubis*.
Scabies: *Sarcoptes scabei*.

Epidemiology

Distribution
- *Pediculosis*: worldwide; head infestation common in children, usually a family infestation; outbreaks occur in schools and institutions: body lice uncommon, usually in vagrants; pubic lice in young adults.
- *Scabies*: worldwide; common in children and young adults; usually a family infestation in conditions of poor hygiene and over-crowding; outbreaks reported in old people's homes and psychiatric hospitals; incidence in population fluctuates with a peak about every 15 years.

Source
- *Pediculosis*: human.
- *Scabies*: human; animal mites do not establish themselves in man.

Spread
- *Pediculosis*: head lice by direct or indirect contact; body lice by direct contact and by clothing and bedding; pubic lice by sexual contact.

Epidemiology

- *Scabies*: direct contact; indirect contact by clothing, bedding and furnishings; sexual transmission.

Pathogenesis
Local damage by parasite aggravated by trauma from scratching and by secondary bacterial infection. Hypersensitivity response to parasite and its products.

Clinical features

Pediculosis
- Head lice may be found anywhere on scalp but tend to concentrate at back of neck. Body lice on any part of body. Pubic lice found in genital area and on eyelashes.
- Intensely itchy red papules and scratch marks.
- Severe and prolonged infestation results in induration and pigmentation of skin (vagabond's disease).
- Secondary bacterial infection common.

Scabies
Rash particularly common around interdigital spaces, on backs of hands, wrists, axillae, groins, breasts, umbilicus, penis and buttocks.
- Severe pruritus aggravated by warmth and moistness.
- Small red slightly elevated papules or vesicles. Typical burrows may not be prominent in clean person.
- Scratching may cause skin damage and result in secondary infection.

Laboratory diagnosis
Scabies mite may be removed from burrow on point of needle and identified by using low-powered lens.

Treatment

Pediculosis
- Malathion lotion or shampoo.
- Carbaryl shampoo.
- Gamma benzene hexachloride application or cream.
- Monosulfiram solution.

Treatment

Scabies
- Benzyl benzoate emulsion: two applications to all members of family.
- Gamma benzene hexachloride 1% cream for children.
- Monosulfiram lotion applied daily for 2–3 days, preferably after hot bath.

Prevention

Immediate — pediculosis
- Isolation: wound precautions in hospital until treated.
- Early treatment of affected child and family.
- Exclusion from school until treated.
- Careful handling and laundering of clothing and bedding in body lice infestation. Steam disinfestation if unsuitable for laundering.

Immediate — scabies
- Isolation: wound precautions in hospital until treated.
- Early effective treatment.
- Case searching and treatment of affected persons in families and institutions.
- Treatment of clothing, bedding and furnishings, as pediculosis above.
- Exclusion from school until treated.

Longterm — pediculosis and scabies
- Avoid contact with infested person.
- Personal hygiene.
- Health education.

Staphylococcal infections

Organisms

Staphylococci: Gram-positive, facultative anaerobes, which grow readily on simple media; two species are of medical importance, *Staph. aureus* and the less virulent *Staph. epidermidis*. Strains of *Staph. aureus* can be recognized by phage typing, which also allows division into four groups (I–IV).

Staph. aureus toxins

- *Coagulase and clumping factors*: two distinct factors, virtually always coexisting, associated with potential pathogenicity but contribution to it obscure; they differentiate *Staph. aureus* (coagulase-positive) and *Staph. epidermidis* (coagulase not produced).
- *Alpha-haemolysin*: antigenic; acts on cell membranes causing lysis, also dermonecrotizing, smooth muscle contracting, haemolytic and lethal; mode of action debated.
- *Delta-haemolysin*: may act synergistically with alpha-haemolysin.
- *Leucocidin*: antigenic; causes altered permeability of polymorphonuclear leucocytes and macrophages.
- *Enterotoxin*: produced by some strains, commonly within phage group III; seven serotypes; activates receptors in gut and reaches vomiting centre via vagus nerve; mechanism of diarrhoea unexplained.
- *Exfoliatin*: most commonly produced by phage group II strains; two serotypes; causes cell separation within epidermis at stratum granulosum (scalded-skin syndrome).
- *Others*: staphylolysin (proteolytic, activating plasminogen to form plasmin), hyaluronidase, lipase, DNase and neuraminidase.

Epidemiology

Distribution

Staph. aureus is a common organism of the skin of man and animals in all parts of the world. In man carriage in anterior nares is present in 36–50% of normal adults but may be as high as 70% in hospital patients; perineal carriage is common; in the neonate colonization of the umbilicus often takes place.

Staphylococcal skin disease is endemic, commonest in warm climates, particularly in children in overcrowded, unhygienic conditions. Wound infections are a frequent manifestation of hospital-acquired infections. Severe staphylococcal disease may occur in highly susceptible persons, such as the elderly following influenza, debilitated and immunocompromised patients in hospitals.

Virulent epidemic strains of *Staph. aureus* may emerge in hospitals associated with use of chemotherapy; in the 1950s and early 1960s a pandemic of staphylococcal disease particularly affecting hospital patients was caused by several strains of antibiotic-resistant *Staph. aureus*, particularly phage type 80/81.

In the late 1970s infections due to a multiple-resistant organism, methicillin-resistant *Staph. aureus* (MRSA), appeared in Europe, North America and Australia, and although less virulent than type 80/81, nevertheless gave rise to serious infections which were difficult to treat because of the limited number of antibiotics to which these strains were sensitive.

An epidemic of staphylococcal shock syndrome took place in the USA in the early 1980s associated with the use of vaginal tampons, over 900 cases in 1980 with 5% mortality. In UK a much lower incidence of fewer than 40 reported cases per year 1982−86, many of them associated with staphylococcal infection at other sites.

Staph. epidermidis, formerly regarded as a non-pathogenic commensal of the skin, gives rise to infections in hospital, particularly in immunocompromised patients and those with prostheses, such as cardiac valves, vascular cannulae and cerebrospinal fluid shunts.

Source
Usually human cases, or nasal or skin carriers.

Spread
Often auto-infection. Spread from discharging staphylococcal lesions, from anterior nares and other sites of asymptomatic carriers by direct or indirect contact. Airborne spread uncommon. Some carriers are particularly prone to disperse staphylococci.

Pathogenesis — *Staph. aureus*
• Pathology of local lesion similar whatever the site. Initial polymorphonuclear response with fluid extravasation; develops into lesion with core of dead cells and bacteria surrounded by fibrin barrier; tension may increase as central liquefaction continues; may heal,

Staphylococcal infections

rupture spontaneously or spread occasionally to surrounding tissues.
- Bacteraemia relatively rare but may be followed by deep abscesses in any organ. Sometimes associated with severe tissue gangrene, presumably due to alpha-toxin.
- Colonization of gastrointestinal tract, following antibiotic-induced disturbance of commensal flora, rare but life-threatening infection.
- Food poisoning due to ingestion of preformed enterotoxin.
- Toxic shock syndrome apparently associated with enterotoxin F; most cases reported in women using tampons during menstruation; *Staph. aureus* recoverable from the vagina.
- Scalded-skin syndrome: see exfoliatin, p. 271.

Pathogenesis — *Staph. epidermidis*
Occasional cause of acute urinary tract infection in young women, otherwise apparently unable to establish infection in normal tissue (but see above). Pathogenetic mechanisms ill understood.

Clinical features — *Staph. aureus*

Skin lesions
- *Impetigo*: bullous lesions common in young children, pustular lesions in older patients.
- *Acute epidermal necrolysis* (scalded skin syndrome): characterized by conjunctivitis, stomatitis, urethritis and a rash; skin extremely painful, large patches of necrotic epidermis slide off the underlying layers leaving extensive raw areas (Nikolsky's sign).
- *Furuncles* and *carbuncles*.
- *Sycosis barbae*.
- *Paronychia*.
- *Cellulitis*.

Surgical sepsis
- *Theatre-acquired infections* generally appear within 3 days of operation.
- *Ward-acquired infections* tend to be more superficial and develop later in convalescence.
- *Stitch abscesses, cellulitis* and *septicaemia*.

Clinical features—*Staph. aureus*

Sepsis in maternity units
- Neonate: pustules and septic bullae, blepharitis and conjunctivitis, breast abscess, pneumonia, septicaemia and osteomyelitis.
- Mother: breast abscess, genital tract sepsis or boils.

Septicaemia
Primary or secondary. Metastatic lesions in bone, heart, kidney and brain.

Food poisoning
See p. 84.

Enterocolitis
Found in elderly debilitated patients recovering from abdominal surgery, especially when treated with broad-spectrum antibiotics. Acute onset of copious diarrhoea, fever and tachycardia ending in circulatory collapse.

Pneumonia
Primary more common in children and starts with upper respiratory symptoms; progresses to pneumonia with increasing respiratory distress; may result in lung abscesses, empyema or pyopneumo-thorax. Secondary may complicate virus infections, such as influenza and chickenpox, or chronic bronchitis and mucoviscidosis.

Toxic shock syndrome
Associated with use of tampons. Fever, erythematous rash, diarrhoea, myalgia accompanied by high blood levels of creatinine phosphokinase, tachycardia and hypotension. Illness may be life-threatening.

Clinical features — *Staph. epidermidis*

Eyes
Marginal blepharitis; keratitis when local immunity is impaired.

Heart
Infection of prostheses.

Clinical features—*Staph. epidermidis*

Brain
Infection of ventriculoatrial or ventriculoperitoneal shunts.

Urinary tract
Acute cystitis in young women.

Systemic infection
Occurs in immunocompromised patients.

Laboratory diagnosis

Culture
- Isolation from pus, or swab in transport medium, taken from accessible lesions usually straightforward.
- *Staph. aureus* identified by coagulase production, sometimes also DNase production; sensitivity testing must be performed for clinical isolates.
- Gram-stained film of pus may aid preliminary diagnosis.
- Blood cultures must be taken in severe illness, or if site of infection inaccessible.
- Culture of suspect food best investigation for food poisoning; isolation from vomitus or stool not regularly successful; tests for enterotoxin production are available.
- Phage typing for epidemiological studies best carried out in a reference laboratory.

Serology
Demonstration of antibodies to the alpha-haemolysin or leucocidin occasionally of assistance in deep-seated infection, but results often disappointing.

Treatment
- Determine sensitivities of organism and select appropriate antibiotic. Benzylpenicillin is antibiotic of choice for sensitive strains.
- Life-threatening infections: high dosage of penicillinase-resistant penicillin i.v. pending results of sensitivity tests. May be supplemented with gentamicin.
- Less severe infections: flucloxacillin orally.

- Trivial infections of skin: local application of antiseptic creams.
- Replace prosthetic valve.
- Replace ventricular shunt if cultures still positive after 10 days' treatment.

Prevention

Immediate
- Isolation: wound/respiratory precautions.
- Report to hospital control-of-infection officer.
- Detection, isolation and treatment of hospital cases and carriers of virulent 'epidemic' strains of *Staph. aureus*.
- Report outbreaks of staphylococcal sepsis in closed communities and schools to health authority to enable investigation and control.

Longterm
- Personal hygiene, handwashing and individual towels in enclosed communities.
- Strict aseptic techniques in hospitals. Meticulous attention to handwashing.
- Hospital antibiotic and disinfectant policies designed to limit the emergence of antibiotic-resistant strains.

Streptococcal infections

The genus *Streptococcus* includes species of medical importance and commensal strains: all are Gram-positive chain-forming cocci — the majority aerobic, a few anaerobic. Beta, alpha and non-haemolytic groups are recognized but the chief differentiation, especially applicable to beta-haemolytic strains, is by characterization of cell-wall polysaccharides (Lancefield grouping): the Lancefield group A organism is *Strep. pyogenes*; other groups include commensal and pathogenic species (e.g. group B, p. 285; group D, enterococci); yet other important species (e.g. *Strep. pneumoniae, Strep. milleri*) cannot be grouped.

1 Group A streptococci (*Strep. pyogenes*)

Organism
Streptococci having the group A cell-wall antigen and other superficial antigens (M, T and R); produce a range of exotoxins.

Toxins
- Streptolysin O: damages cells by binding to cholesterol in membranes; cardiotoxic for many animals, possibly including man; potent antigen.
- Streptolysin S: also a haemolysin but mode of action not understood; toxic to leucocytes; not antigenic.
- Deoxyribonuclease (streptodornase), streptokinase, hyaluronidase: all probably contribute to spread of infection through tissues.
- Erythrogenic toxins: produced by some strains; three serotypes, A, B and C; antigenic.

M, T and R antigens
Superficial, protein antigens; characterized for epidemiological studies. M antigens important virulence factors, induce type-specific immunity; certain types recognized as nephritogenic.

Epidemiology

Distribution
Common infection in temperate zones, highest incidence in winter in

children. Pharyngitis, sore throat and scarlet fever commonest clinical manifestations of infection. Often symptomless, up to 20% of children may be pharyngeal carriers. Streptococcal disease has fallen in incidence and severity in past 40 years; this is probably associated with a natural decline in virulence of the organism. In UK notifications of scarlet fever declined from over 80 000 per year in 1940s to fewer than 8000 in 1980s.

Erysipelas, more frequent in adults than children, and puerperal sepsis (see p. 222), have also declined. Streptococcal impetigo affects mainly young children living in poor hygienic conditions, seasonal peak in late summer. Rheumatic fever and acute glomerulonephritis now uncommon in UK; hospital in-patients with rheumatic fever fell from over 3500 in 1957 to fewer than 400 in 1986, and with acute nephritis from about 2700 in 1957 to about 1000 in 1986. In USA a similar fall in streptococcal disease was seen until 1986, when a resurgence of acute rheumatic fever with several localized outbreaks was reported associated with infections caused by mucoid strains of *Strep. pyogenes*.

Source
Human: infected respiratory secretions, septic skin lesions. Occasionally cattle.

Spread
Direct contact with infected respiratory secretions. Indirect contact by hands. Airborne droplets. Foodborne and sometimes milkborne.

Pathogenesis

Acute infections
Site of entry, e.g. throat, skin or elsewhere, governs the type of disease; extension into surrounding tissues may be rapid, as may spread into lymphatics and bloodstream.
Scarlet fever: erythrogenic toxins responsible for skin capillary damage, possibly also for pyrexia and may potentiate other streptococcal toxins. Antibodies from previous contact with erythrogenic toxins prevent rash in any subsequent infection.

Pathogenesis

Late sequelae
Immunologically based, probably type II hypersensitivity reactions; rheumatic fever occurs in predisposed individuals, recurring on subsequent infection with another M type; glomerulonephritis associated with relatively few M types, repeated attacks are therefore rare.

Clinical features — streptococcal tonsillitis

Incubation period
Usually 2–4 days.

Older children and adults
Sudden onset of sore throat accompanied by general disturbance with fever, headache and malaise. Fauces inflamed, tonsils swollen and patches of whitish exudate present in about half of patients. Tonsillar lymph nodes enlarged and tender. Duration of illness short.

Infants and children under 3 years
Focal signs less prominent. Low-grade fever and prolonged course. Seldom exudate. Vomiting and abdominal pain.

Clinical features — scarlet fever

Incubation period
Usually 2–4 days.

Onset
Abrupt with fever, sore throat, headache and malaise. Sore throat may be absent in children but vomiting is common.

Throat
Painful especially on swallowing. Tonsils inflamed and swollen; may be covered with patchy or confluent white exudate. Fauces and palate reddened and stippled.

Tongue
• *'White strawberry' stage*: coated with white fur through which the enlarged papillae stand out.

Clinical features—scarlet fever

- *'Red strawberry' stage*: white fur peels from the edges and tips inwards leaving prominent papillae on glazed surface.

Rash
After 24 hours a bright flush appears on the face sparing the lips (circumoral pallor), then spreads rapidly over the body and limbs. Punctate erythema on trunk and discrete fine macules on distal parts of limbs. Rash heavy in hollows. Fades from above downwards and disappears within a week. Desquamation starts over clavicles about fourth or fifth day of rash and gradually extends to the hands and feet by end of second week.

Cervical lymph nodes
Swollen and tender.

Complications
- Septic: rhinitis, sinusitis and otitis media; suppurative lymphadenitis.
- Immunological reactions: rheumatic fever and nephritis.

Other forms
- Surgical scarlet fever from infected wounds or burns.
- Infected chickenpox lesions.
- Puerperal scarlet fever.

Clinical features — erysipelas

Incubation period
Less than 1 week.

Onset
Abrupt with headache, malaise, vomiting and pyrexia.

Local lesion
Appears within a few hours. Raised, tense, rapidly spreading area of erythema with sharply defined palpable edge. Bullae common. Rash fades leaving staining. Frequently accompanied by cellulitis.

Clinical features—erysipelas

Common sites
Face, especially butterfly-wing distribution. Leg.

Complications
Local abscesses, septicaemia and persistent lymphoedema of legs.

Other syndromes
- Impetigo.
- Cellulitis, lymphangitis and lymphadenitis.
- Otitis media and sinusitis.
- Post-abortum and post-partum sepsis (see p. 222).
- Septicaemia.
- Pneumonia: usually follows virus infection.

Treatment — acute *Strep. pyogenes* infection
- Mild attack of scarlet fever or tonsillitis in area with low incidence of rheumatic fever: symptomatic treatment, no antibiotics.
- Severe attack or attack in area with high incidence of rheumatic fever: benzylpenicillin i.m. followed by phenoxymethylpenicillin orally; erythromycin for patients hypersensitive to penicillin.
- Eradication of streptococcus from nasopharynx: phenoxymethyl penicillin orally for minimum of 10 days or benzathine penicillin 916 mg i.m. single dose.
- Benzylpenicillin or erythromycin for treatment of erysipelas and other severe infections.
- Consider elastic stocking for prevention of lymphoedema after erysipelas of leg.

Clinical features — rheumatic fever

Onset
History of sore throat 10–21 days previously in 70%. In children illness starts insidiously with lassitude, malaise and vague joint and muscle pains; in adults onset is abrupt with sharp rise in temperature followed immediately by pain in one or more joints.

Fever
Intermittent or remittent, seldom exceeds 39°C. Good index of activity.

Arthritis
Classically migratory. Mainly large joints. Severity very variable. May be absent, especially in children.

Heart
Tachycardia is the rule. Carditis if one or more of following: diastolic or loud systolic murmurs, pericarditis, cardiac enlargement or congestive heart failure. About two-thirds of children with rheumatic fever eventually develop chronic rheumatic heart disease.

Skin
Erythematous rashes. Subcutaneous nodules, especially in children.

Nervous system
About 10% of patients subsequently develop chorea.

Course
Prolonged illness with frequent relapses.

Treatment — rheumatic fever
- Bedrest until all signs of activity have subsided: normal temperature, WBC, ESR and no signs of carditis.
- Salicylates or acetylsalicylic acid until symptom-free and nornal ESR.
- Prednisolone for carditis with heart failure.
- Chemoprophylaxis: benzathine penicillin 916 mg i.m. every 3 weeks, or phenoxymethylpenicillin 125 mg orally daily, or sulphadimidine or sulphadiazine 1 g orally daily (see p. 343).

Clinical features — acute glomerulonephritis

Glomerular filtration
Impaired. Salt and water retention, mild generalized oedema and hypertension.

Clinical features—acute glomerulonephritis

Urine
Slight to moderate proteinuria, less than 5 g/24 hours. Microscopic or macroscopic haematuria. Deposit shows red blood cells, red blood cell and granular casts and occasionally white blood cell casts.

Circulation
Expansion in blood volume with elevation of jugular venous pressure. Variable hypertension. Bradycardia.

Nephrotic syndrome
Develops in small proportion but is transient.

Complications
Hypertensive encephalopathy, pulmonary oedema and acute renal failure.

Prognosis
Excellent in children. Small amounts of protein, cells or casts may persist for long periods in adults.

Treatment — acute glomerulonephritis
- Bedrest during acute phase.
- Short course of benzylpenicillin.
- Salt restriction, diuretics and antihypertensive drugs.

Laboratory diagnosis — *Strep. pyogenes* infection

Culture
- Nose and throat swabs or pus must be collected before starting antibiotic treatment. Blood cultures should be taken if infection inaccessible, if rapidly extending or if patient very ill.
- Recovery of *Strep. pyogenes* may not be successful from patients with rheumatic fever or other late sequelae but should be attempted.
- Isolation of *Strep. pyogenes* usually straightforward but selective media helpful for specimens from sites with heavy commensal flora. Screening of primary culture possible with bacitracin sensitivity discs (diagnostic strength) but definitive identification is by detection of

group A antigen by precipitation, coagglutination or immunofluorescent methods.
- Antibiotic sensitivity should be confirmed, especially if erythromycin is prescribed.

Serology
Elevated titre of antibodies against streptolysin O (ASO) indicates recent streptococcal infection (virtually always with *Strep. pyogenes*). In UK healthy schoolchildren rarely have titres >200 u, adults usually lower. Titres >200 u usual in 60–70% of patients with rheumatic fever and glomerulonephritis.

Prevention — *Strep. pyogenes* infection

Immediate
- Isolation: respiratory/wound precautions.
- Specific chemotherapy.
- Report to health authority outbreaks of streptococcal infection for investigation and control.
- Scarlet fever notifiable in UK.
- Exclude from work or school until clinical recovery.
- In hospital outbreaks inform control-of-infection officer.
- Nose and throat swabs of close contacts in maternity units and other special circumstances.
- Treatment of carriers: see above.

Longterm
- Early effective treatment of streptococcal infections.
- Food hygiene, pasteurization of milk.
- Strict asepsis in obstetric and hospital practice.
- Continuous chemoprophylaxis of patients with rheumatic fever throughout childhood to prevent recurrence.

2 Group B streptococci

Organism
Streptococci having the group B antigen (*Strep. agalactiae*): further typing using superficial protein antigens useful epidemiologically. Majority of strains non-haemolytic; other toxins not prominent.

Epidemiology

Distribution
An important cause of neonatal and infant bacteraemia and meningitis, first recognized in late 1950s and early 1960s, may be increasing in incidence, probably about 0.3 per 1000 live births in UK. Carrier rates of 5–25% in genital tracts of normal women in late pregnancy, carrier rates may be higher in non-pregnant women. The organism may also be found in anorectal area.

In UK over 150 cases of bacteraemia and meningitis reported annually in infants in 1985–87 and about twice this number of infections in older age groups, most frequently adults over 45 years. High mortality in early neonatal cases, usually associated with low birth weight, prolonged interval between rupture of the membranes and birth, and maternal genital tract infection.

Source
Human.

Spread
Early neonatal infection probably from infected birth canal; late neonatal infection probably arises by nosocomial spread.

Pathogenesis
Processes not well understood: evidence suggests that severe infection occurs in patients deficient in type-specific opsonizing antibody. Predisposition in neonates of low birth weight and after prolonged membrane rupture. Associated conditions in adults include diabetes, reticuloendothelial diseases, pregnancy and gynaecological operations.

Clinical features — neonatal infection

Early onset
- Usually within first 3 days after birth.
- Usually associated with prematurity or difficult birth.
- Generalized sepsis resulting in poor general condition, failure to feed, lethargy, irritability and poor activity.
- Respiratory distress with cyanosis and periods of apnoea. Chest X-ray suggests hyaline-membrane disease.
- Bacteraemia common; one-third develop meningitis.
- Mortality over 50%.

Late onset
- After first week — usually around fourth week.
- Onset less acute and illness less severe.
- Bacteraemia very common; meningitis 75%.
- Pulmonary involvement rare.
- Neonatal sepsis may involve many structures.
- Asymptomatic bacteraemia in a few.
- Mortality 20%. Residual damage to CNS common in survivors.

Clinical features — adult infection
- Obstetric or gynaecological procedures in previously healthy young women — pelvic sepsis, bacteraemia.
- Patients of 60 years and older with serious disease, especially diabetes complicated by peripheral vascular disease — bacteraemia, endocarditis and meningitis. Also pulmonary and renal tract infections.

Laboratory diagnosis

Culture
- *Neonates*: blood culture, CSF, throat swab, gastric aspirate, and specimens from other sites, to detect superficial colonization, should be examined without delay.
- *Adults*: blood cultures and specimens from other sites as indicated clinically. Selective media should be used for specimens from sites with commensal flora: group B streptococci are bile tolerant and will

grow on simple bile-containing media (e.g. MacConkey's medium); growth on bile-aesculin medium, but without hydrolysis of aesculin, is a useful preliminary test; definitive identification is by detection of the group antigen.

Treatment
- Benzylpenicillin.
- Benzylpenicillin in combination with an aminoglycoside.
- Group B streptococci are all sensitive to cephalosporins and to chloramphenicol.

Prevention

Immediate
- Isolation; wound precautions.
- Inform hospital control-of-infection officer, especially in late neonatal onset, so that source of infection may be traced and controlled.

Longterm
- High standards of antenatal and obstetric care.
- Hospital infection control measures.
- Chemoprophylaxis with penicillin has been suggested for bacteriologically-positive mothers and neonates. Chemoprophylaxis has also been suggested for high-risk neonates, such as premature babies and those born after early rupture of membranes.

3 Other species of streptococci

Group C streptococci
Found in throat of healthy individuals; may cause sore throats. Food-borne infection has been reported. *Strep. zooepidemicus*, a species within group C, may cause septic infections in persons associated with cattle. Milkborne outbreaks have been reported causing bacteraemia and meningitis with high mortality in the elderly.

Faecal streptococci (group D)
Streptococci of Lancefield group D, including *Strep. faecalis, faecium,*

bovis and *durans*; haemolysis varies from strain to strain; bile tolerant intestinal commensals. Low-grade pathogens; responsible for some urinary tract infections and infections of wounds or skin ulcers; important role in infective endocarditis, especially following gynaecological operations or urinary tract instrumentation (see p. 73–6); less sensitive to benzylpenicillin than other *Streptococcus* spp.

Group L streptococci
Cause infection in dogs, pigs, cattle and sheep. Skin infections have been reported in meat and animal handlers; infected wounds, impetigo and paronychia, sometimes in association with *Staph. aureus*.

Group R streptococci
Streptococcus suis type 2 causes infection in pigs and was first reported giving rise to bacteraemia and meningitis in pig handlers in UK in 1976, fewer than 20 cases reported in UK 1976–86.

Viridans streptococci
A heterogeneous group, including *Strep. viridans, milleri, mitior, mutans, salivarius* and *sanguis*; alpha-haemolytic; commensals of mouth and pharynx. Low-grade pathogens but important in infective endocarditis (see p. 73) and some species, especially *Strep. mutans*, have a role in dental caries.

Anaerobic streptococci (peptococci, peptostreptococci) and microaerophilic streptococci
A large group including many species, not all well characterized; commensals of mucous membranes. Commonly isolated, often with other anaerobes, from clinical material, probably contributing to disease process: undoubtedly pathogenic in some situations, e.g. post-abortum and post-partum infection (see p. 222) anaerobic cellulitis and myositis (may mimic clostridial infection), synergistic bacterial gangrene of the skin and occasionally in endocarditis (p. 74)

Streptococcus pneumoniae
A capsulated, aerobic diplococcus; commensal in upper respiratory tract. Identified by sensitivity to Optochin (ethylhydrocuprein-hydrochloride) or by bile solubility. Virulent toxins not produced.

Streptococcal infections: Other species

Streptococcus pneumoniae

The polysaccharide capsule is antiphagocytic; specific opsonizing antibodies and complement are necessary for phagocytosis and killing. More than 80 serotypes recognized, the 14 most common accounting for 70−80% of pneumococcal pneumonias; in UK type 3 isolated from 20−25% and, types 1, 4, 6, 7 and 8, from 60% (see p. 214). Distribution of serotypes differs in infants and older age groups and there is some variation worldwide.

Important pathogen in meningitis (see pp. 178−81), also responsible for some cases of otitis media, conjunctivitis and peritonitis.

Tetanus

Organism
Clostridium tetani: Gram-positive spore-bearing anaerobic rod which produces a potent exotoxin.

Epidemiology

Distribution
Worldwide, high incidence in neonates in Africa, Asia and South America; rare in countries with effective routine infant immunization programmes and high standards of care of wounded. May occur in injecting drug abusers. In UK disease declining, probably fewer than 30 cases per year 1980—87, almost none under 15 years of age; more common in young adult men than women, but in the elderly it is more common in women because of immunization of men on military service; 1—2 deaths per year reported. In 1980s five unrelated cases reported in UK with an apparent association with gallbladder surgery.

Source
Widely distributed in soil, dust and gastrointestinal tracts of animals.

Spread
Direct introduction of spores by penetrating injury. Direct contamination of wounds, burns, umbilical stumps by dust or faeces. Contaminated syringes used by drugs addicts. No person-to-person transmission.

Pathogenesis
Germination of spores occurs when introduced into tissues with low oxygen tension, e.g. wounds with necrotic tissue including those with concomitant contamination with aerobic bacteria. Exotoxin, produced only by vegetative organisms, is taken up by local motor-nerve endings, travels within axons to spinal cord, and is released from motor neurone. At the synapse toxin blocks action of the inhibitory neurone thus causing tetanic spasm. The organism itself is not invasive.

Clinical features

Incubation period
Usually 7−10 days, extremes 18 hours to 2.5 years.

Prodromal period
Restlessness, irritability and malaise for 24 hours.

Hypertonus
Trismus and neck stiffness followed in few hours by rigidity of trunk muscles. Facial spasm produces risus sardonicus. In severe attack tonic rigidity at peak within a day or two; mild cases advance slowly for several weeks.

Reflex spasms
Violent sustained contraction of all somatic muscles. Frequency and severity variable. Patient remains fully conscious. Spasms cease after 7−21 days leaving hypertonus for 2−3 months. Death from exhaustion, asphyxia or inhalation pneumonia. Autonomic nervous system may be affected.

Special varieties
Neonatal, puerperal, local, cephalic, otogenic, splanchnic and modified.

Prognosis
Grave with incubation period less than 7 days or interval to first spasms less than 24 hours; favourable with incubation period greater than 14 days or interval to paroxysm exceeding 3 days.

Laboratory diagnosis
Clinical diagnosis paramount; laboratory diagnosis may be difficult, especially if the site of infection is small. If available, pus in a sterile container is preferable to swab in transport medium.

Microscopy
Gram-positive or Gram-variable rods with round, terminal spores; usually scanty, may not be demonstrable; not pathognomonic.

Tetanus

Laboratory diagnosis

Anaerobic culture
Swarming growth; recognition of *Clostridium tetani* may be time consuming as mixed anaerobic infections may occur; final indentification by inoculation into two mice, one of which is protected with antitoxin.

Treatment

Antitoxin
Human tetanus immunoglobulin 30−300 iu/kg bodyweight or equine antitoxin 10 000−20 000 u by i.m. injection.

Antibiotics
Benzylpenicillin i.m. in mild attacks, i.v. in severe cases.

Surgery
Indicated to remove foreign matter, excise necrotic tissue and restore blood supply whenever possible. Antitoxin should be given at least 1 hour previously.

Sedation
Phenobarbitone, amylobarbitone, diazepam and chlorpromazine singly or in combination.

Tracheostomy and curarization
In a sedated patient one spasm is indication for tracheostomy and insertion of cuffed tube. If further spasm interferes with breathing the patient should be paralysed and artificially ventilated.

Prevention

Immediate — tetanus case
- Isolation: unnecessary.
- Report to health authority; notifiable in UK.
- Investigation of source of infection.
- Active immunization concurrent with specific therapy.

Immediate — tetanus exposure
- Chemoprophylaxis with parenteral penicillin, followed by oral

Tetanus

Prevention

penicillin, commencing before surgical toilet and continued for 5 days; alternatively erythromycin or metronidazole.
- Surgical toilet of wound.
- Assessment of risk of tetanus by type and extent of wound, degree of contamination, length of time elapsing between injury and surgical toilet, secondary infection and history of immunization against tetanus.

- Immunization after tetanus exposure

Type of wound	History of immunization with tetanus toxoid			
	Primary course with or without reinforcing dose			None, incomplete or not known
	<5 years	5–10 years before	10+ years before	
Minor, superficial, sustained within previous 6 hours	None	Toxoid reinforcing dose	Toxoid reinforcing dose	Toxoid* first dose
Sustained over 6 hours previously. Clean, moderate tissue damage or penetrating	None	Toxoid reinforcing dose	Toxoid reinforcing dose HTIG	Toxoid* first dose HTIG
Neglected, contaminated, secondarily infected or severe tissue damage	Toxoid reinforcing dose HTIG	Toxoid reinforcing dose HTIG	Toxoid reinforcing dose HTIG	Toxoid* first dose HTIG

* Adsorbed tetanus vaccine (Tet/Vac/Ads) 0.5 ml, second dose 6–12 weeks later, third dose 4–12 months later.
HTIG = human tetanus immunoglobulin 250–500 u i.m.

Tetanus

Longterm
- Tetanus prevention in the wounded (see above).
- Routine active immunization in childhood (p. 357).
- Health education in care of umbilical stump to prevent neonatal tetanus.
- Immunization of pregnant women to confer passive immunity to the newborn in countries with high incidence of tetanus.

Toxoplasmosis

Organism

Toxoplasma gondii: protozoan first recognized in the gondi, a North African rodent, but capable of infecting a wide range of animals. Sexual cycle takes place in the cat which is probably infected by ingesting birds and small rodents; toxoplasmas develop in gastro-intestinal tract mucosa, forming long-surviving faecal oocysts. Man infected either by ingestion of oocysts or of tissue cysts from raw meat. In man the proliferative form is the crescent-shaped trophozoite, which becomes encysted in the resting phase.

Epidemiology

Distribution
Worldwide zoonosis, unevenly distributed with particularly high inci-dence in Central America and France. Common infection but clinical disease rare. In UK about half adults aged 50 years have antibody; about 700 laboratory-reported cases per year 1975−86 with one to two registered deaths; about 62% cases presented with eye disease, 27% with glandular disease and 4% with congenital disease. Con-genital infection in about 40% of infants born to mothers primarily infected during pregnancy; most infected infants develop clinical disease; lowest risk of transmission in early pregnancy, but severest disease. Frequent manifestation of Aids, giving rise to infection of brain and nervous system, particularly in Africa.

Source
The cat is a definitive host, and excretes oocysts in stools which infect other animals on ingestion. Infection widespread in food animals, such as sheep, pigs, goats and cattle.

Spread
Human infection occurs by eating raw or undercooked infected meat, by eating vegetables contaminated with infected soil or by the inges-tion of oocysts excreted in cat faeces. Waterborne and milkborne (goat) outbreaks have been described.

Pathogenesis

Fetal infection
Placental transfer of organism following parasitaemia during maternal primary infection; most severe effects on fetus during first trimester; latent maternal infection not usually transmitted.

Acquired infection
Toxoplasmas, presumably following ingestion of organism and subsequent parasitaemia, invade and multiply within endothelial cells; released by cell rupture. Apparent predilection for nervous tissue. In acute infections toxoplasmas may be demonstrable singly or in pairs; in chronic infection multicellular cysts found, no true capsule but surrounding host-tissue reaction forms apparent capsule.

Clinical features

Congenital
- Abortion, miscarriage or stillbirth.
- Classical triad: hydrocephalus, cerebral calcification and chorioretinitis in 60%.
- Eye damage: chorioretinitis, uveitis, cataracts and panophthalmitis. Late features: nystagmus, squints and retinal detachment.
- CNS: microcephaly, retardation, epilepsy, cerebral calcification, hydrocephalus.
- Other features: splenomegaly, hepatomegaly and jaundice, anaemia, rashes, pneumonitis.

Acquired
- Benign lymphadenitis resembling infectious mononucleosis.
- Chorioretinitis.
- Encephalitis.
- Typhus-like illness: high fever, rashes and pneumonitis. Usually fatal.

Laboratory diagnosis

Serology
Humoral antibodies detectable by Sabin−Feldman dye test, passive
haemagglutination or fluorescent methods, the last permitting
differentiation of IgM and IgG responses.
- *Acute infection*: fluorescent (IgM) and dye tests become positive
early; passive haemagglutination antibodies appear later; rising titre
should be demonstrable.
- *Subclinical infection*: approximately 30% of UK population have
antibody detectable at low titre (up to 200 iu) indicating previous
clinical or subclinical infection.
- *Chronic focal infection* (e.g. ocular toxoplasmosis): antibody titres
indistinguishable from subclinical infection: IgM response not
demonstrable.

Culture
Isolation from blood or body fluids by culture in eggs, or inoculation
of mice is possible, but serological diagnosis more common.
Trophozoites or cysts may occasionally be demonstrable histologically in biopsy material.

Treatment
- Unnecessary in mild infections.
- Pyrimethamine 25−50 mg and sulphadimidine 4−8 g daily for
2−4 weeks.
- Spiramycin 2−4 g daily for 2−6 weeks.
- Prednisolone in combination with pyrimethamine and sulpha-
dimidine for eye infection.

Prevention

Immediate
- Isolation: unnecessary.
- Search for possible associated cases.
- Report clusters to health authority for investigation and control of
source of infection.
- Infection in pregnancy: consider therapeutic abortion.

Toxoplasmosis

Prevention

Longterm
- Avoid undercooked or raw meat, especially during pregnancy or in immunocompromised.
- Handwashing after gardening and after handling raw vegetables.
- Careful hygiene when disposing of cat excreta.
- Pasteurization of milk.

Treponemal infections

1 Syphilis

Organism

Treponema pallidum: a human parasitic spirochaete; invisible by routine microscopy; best seen by dark-ground illumination. Culture in artificial media and tissue cells not yet possible; sensitive to drying, dies rapidly above 42°C, but survives some days at 4°C (e.g. in refrigerated blood). Indistinguishable morphologically or by serology from treponemes causing yaws, pinta and bejel. Other species (e.g. *T. microdentium*) are commensals.

Epidemiology

Distribution
Worldwide, primary infection commonest in young adults. Increased in many countries in 1960s and 70s, less marked in UK, and mainly in homosexual males. Decrease in homosexually acquired male syphilis noted in many countries in mid 1980s following publicity about mode of spread of Aids, but heterosexually acquired infection in young adults increased. Congenital syphilis rare in countries with declining incidence of syphilis and effective antenatal screening programmes; in UK one to nine cases per year 1980–86.

Source
Human.

Spread
Sexual contact. Direct contact with moist lesions of skin or mucous membranes. Fetal infection via placenta.

Pathogenesis

Acquired infection
Primary lesion at site of implantation; organism extends to regional lymph nodes and thence to the bloodstream, causing widespread infection in secondary stage. Skin and mucous membrane lesions of secondary stage highly infectious. Even untreated, secondary lesions heal; relatively few treponemes survive into subsequent stages.

Pathogenesis

Granulomatous lesions of tertiary stage excessive in view of scanty organisms; hypersensitivity probably contributory.

Congenital infection
Secondary stage disease in mother affects fetus causing abortion, stillbirth, neonatal death, or a wide range of developmental abnormalities.

Clinical features

Incubation period
Extremes 9−90 days; usually 21−35 days.

Clinical features — primary syphilis

Primary chancre
Genital site 90%; commonest extragenital site the anal canal. Single lesion 50%. Evolves rapidly from macule to papule, which erodes and forms round painless ulcer with clean surface and surrounding hard induration. Heals within 3−10 weeks.

Regional lymph nodes
Swollen 50%; discrete, rubbery, relatively painless. Suppuration only if secondarily infected.

Clinical features — secondary syphilis

Skin lesions
Initial presentation in 70% of cases, usually 6−8 weeks after infection. Characteristically pleomorphic, symmetrical and generalized. Rash varies greatly in intensity and appearance. Mild alopecia common.

Mucous patches
Round, greyish-white, slightly raised patch on mucous membranes, which undergoes erosion or ulceration. Highly infectious. Found in mouth, pharynx, larynx or genital organs concurrently with skin rash.

Other features
Lymphadenitis, meningitis, periostitis, hepatitis and iridocyclitis.

General symptoms
Fever headache, malaise, anorexia, and arthralgia.

Clinical features — latent syphilis
Begins when secondary stage subsides. No clinical evidence of active disease but serological tests remain positive.

Tertiary syphilis
Between 10 and 40% of patients with latent syphilis develop tertiary syphilis 3–10 years or longer after infection. The basic lesion is a chronic granuloma, known as a gumma, which tends to be localized, asymmetrical in distribution and destructive in character.

Skin lesions
Nodulocutaneous syphilide and squamous tertiary syphilide. Subcutaneous gumma begins as a painless swelling in the deep tissues and breaks down to form a punched-out ulcer. Healing produces characteristic tissue-paper scarring.

Bone lesions
Osteoporosis and subperiosteal deposition of new bone. Symptomless or gnawing boring pain. Local swelling of bone. History of trauma.

Cardiovascular lesions
Aortitis, coronary ostial stenosis, aortic aneurysm and aortic regurgitation. Appears 10–30 years after infection. About 30% have concomitant neurosyphilis.

Neurosyphilis
Now rare. Meningovascular syphilis appears about 3–7 years after infection, general paralysis of the insane about 10 years after, and tabes dorsalis 15–20 years after infection.

Clinical features — congenital syphilis
Now a great rarity in developed countries.

Clinical features—congenital syphilis

Early manifestations
Osteochondritis and periostitis. Rhinitis. Rash. Fissures and mucous patches. Fever. Anaemia, haemorrhages and splenomegaly. Hepatomegaly and jaundice. Loss of hair and nails. Choroiditis and iritis.

Late manifestations
Damage to teeth, bones, eyes and auditory nerve. Gummata. Neurosyphilis.

Laboratory diagnosis — primary syphilis
● Demonstration of *T. pallidum* by dark-ground microscopy of exudate from chancre; confusion with commensal treponemes, especially in oral lesions, possible in inexperienced hands.
● Serology unlikely to be positive early in primary stage (fluorescent treponemal antibody usually first positive test) but baseline serological test should be performed to gauge success of therapy.

Laboratory diagnosis — post-primary syphilis
Confirmatory diagnosis dependent on serological tests, of which there are two main types: reaginic and specific.

Reaginic tests
Non-specific, cardiolipid antigen; chief tests are:
● VDRL (Venereal Disease Research Laboratory).
● RPR (rapid plasma reagin).
● ART (automated reagin test).
Useful for indicating activity of disease (titre falls rapidly after treatment of early infection). Biological false-positive reactions may occur with autoimmune diseases, with some acute infections, and sometimes in pregnancy. Positive findings must be confirmed with specific tests.

Specific tests
T. pallidum antigens; chief tests are:
● TPHA (*T. pallidum* haemagglutination).
● FTA.Abs (fluorescent treponemal antibody, absorbed).
● TPI (*T. pallidum* immobilization).
Used for confirmation of diagnosis. Little value in following success

of treatment (titre may fall slowly after successful treatment, or may remain positive for years despite adequate therapy).

● Initial positive findings should always be confirmed on a second specimen.

● Impossible to distinguish between syphilis and other treponemal infections serologically.

Laboratory diagnosis — congenital syphilis

● Maternal serology will be positive.

● Active infection in infant (rather than transplacental transfer of maternal antibody) confirmed by demonstrating IgM class antibodies in cord blood.

Treatment

● Procaine penicillin: 600 mg i.m. daily for 10−21 days according to stage of infection.

● Oxytetracycline, erythromycin or cephaloridine should be considered for patients hypersensitive to penicillin.

● Follow-up monthly for 3 months then 3-monthly for 18 months with clinical examination and reagin blood tests. Lumbar puncture during second year.

● Avoid sexual relations for at least 1 year following treatment.

Prevention

Immediate

● Isolation: wound precautions for primary and secondary syphilis until treated.

● Report to STD clinic or health authority.

● Early specific treatment and follow-up.

● Identification of contacts, their investigation and if necessary treatment.

Longterm

● Health education.

● Detection and early treatment of infectious cases.

● Antenatal serological screening and treatment if required.

2 Yaws

Organism
Treponema pertenue: indistinguishable from *T. pallidum*: neither organism can be cultured and thus their relationships cannot be determined.

Epidemiology

Distribution
Tropical and subtropical countries, mainly rural areas. Highest incidence in children in poor economic circumstances, commoner in males than females.

Source
Human.

Spread
Direct contact with lesions of infected person.

Pathogenesis
Primary lesion presumed to occur at site of inoculation of treponemes; penetration probably aided by minor skin trauma. Course of subsequent infection bears many similarities to syphilis.

Clinical features

Incubation period
Usually 3−6 weeks.

Clinical features — primary stage

Primary lesion
Site varies but commonly lower limb or buttocks. Initial lesion, an erythematous macule, develops into an exuberant granulomatous papule 20−40 mm in diameter. Serous exudate from damaged epithelial covering forms yellowish scab. Heals after 3−4 months.

Clinical features — secondary stage

Skin lesions

About 3 months after primary lesions multiple secondary lesions emerge on any part of the skin and particularly around mucocutaneous junctions. Yaw papules vary in size from 5–20 mm in diameter, occasionally much larger, and may be surmounted by a yellowish crust. Itchy but not painful except on palms and soles, where lesions are deeply embedded and associated with hyperkeratosis. Maximum size is attained after 2 weeks and they heal spontaneously in a few months. Mucous membranes not affected. Successive crops months or years apart. Lymph nodes enlarged with secondary infection.

Bone lesions

Multiple areas of osteitis and periostitis involving particularly the long bones of forearms and legs. Dactylitis especially troublesome in children. Deposition of new bone around the nose produces severe facial deformity known as goundou. Bone lesions develop and resolve rapidly; relapses common.

Clinical features — tertiary stage

Skin lesions

Similar to nodulocutaneous syphilides. Gummatous lesions may ulcerate deeply, especially when secondarily infected, causing much deformity. May progress directly from earlier stages or develop many years after secondary lesions have healed. Depigmented patches on hands, feet and ankles are characteristic.

Bone lesions

Fewer bones involved than in secondary stage. Osteoporosis, necrosis and new bone formation. Leads to hideous deformities, especially of face (gangosa). Sabre-shaped deformity of tibia known as boomerang leg.

Juxta-articular nodes
Firm, painless, subcutaneous, fibrous tumours, about the size of a small orange, near large joints. Characteristic feature of late yaws.

Laboratory diagnosis
The serological findings and their response to treatment are as in syphilis (see p. 302). Adults treated in childhood for yaws would be expected to have positive specific tests, but absent or low levels of antibody in non-specific tests.

Treatment
Procaine penicillin in oil with 2% aluminium monostearate.

Individual treatment
Two i.m. injections separated by an interval of 3−5 days. Total adult dosage 1.2 g; children 5−15 years 600 mg; children under 5 years 125 mg.

Mass treatment
Adults and older children a single injection of 600 mg; children under 5 years 125 mg. Follow-up essential.

Prevention

Immediate
- Isolation: wound precautions until treated.
- Report to STD clinic or health authority.
- Early specific treatment.
- Identification and treatment of close contacts.

Longterm
- Improvement in hygiene in endemic areas.
- Health education.
- Population control programmes by mass clinical screening and treatment of cases (see above).

Tularaemia

Organism
Francisella tularensis: small Gram-negative rod, previously named
Pasteurella tularensis. Antigenically homogeneous but varies in viru-
lence and sensitivity to antibiotics.

Epidemiology

Distribution
Confined to northern hemisphere: reported in continental Europe,
North America and Japan; usually sporadic, occasional outbreaks
reported.

Source
Wild animals, especially rabbits and hares.

Spread
Direct handling of infected animals; tick-borne; foodborne due to
eating inadequately cooked contaminated meat; waterborne; airborne,
particularly in laboratories. Not transmitted from person to person.

Pathogenesis
Local infection at site of entry and spread via lymphatics to bloodstream.

Clinical features
- Incubation 2 – 10 days.
- Frequently asymptomatic.
- Usually discharging ulcer at portal of entry: skin, eye or mouth.
May be absent, or may be trivial and sole manifestation.
- Lymphangitis and regional lymphadenitis.
- Typhoidal state associated with severe general symptoms and
high fever.
- Pneumonia, septicaemia or meningitis.

Laboratory diagnosis
- Serological: agglutinating antibodies appear towards the end of
the first week and rise to high titres.
- Culture of discharges is hazardous and should only be carried out
in specialized laboratories.

Treatment
- Streptomycin is drug of choice: 30−40 mg/kg/day. Gentamicin has also proved effective.
- Tetracycline or chloramphenicol by mouth may be used to complete the course of antibiotic therapy once the acute stage has subsided.

Prevention

Immediate
- Isolation: unnecessary once diagnosis has been established.
- Report to health authority for epidemiological investigation.
- Search for other cases possibly exposed to same source of infection.

Longterm
- Avoid contact with potentially infected animals.
- Impervious gloves when handling or skinning animals.
- Avoid drinking or immersion in untreated water in endemic areas.
- Scrupulous care in handling laboratory specimens.
- Immunization of persons at special risk.

Typhus

Organisms

Species of rickettsiae: small Gram-negative coccobacilli; obligate intracellular parasites; multiply by binary fission; contain both nucleic acids; sensitive to several antibacterial antibiotics. Vectorborne. Species differentiation by antigenic analysis. Of chief importance: *Rickettsia prowazeki*, epidemic louse-borne typhus; *R. typhi*, murine typhus; *R. rickettsii*, Rocky Mountain spotted fever; *R. tsutsugamushi*, scrub typhus.

Epidemiology

Distribution

● *Louse-borne (classical epidemic typhus)*: distributed worldwide and occurs where poor, overcrowded, unhygienic living conditions promote the spread of infestation with body lice. Now endemic in parts of Asia, Africa, Central and South America.

● *Flea-borne (murine endemic typhus)*: distributed worldwide but localized in areas of heavy rat infestation, particularly parts of Africa and South America.

● *Tick-borne typhus (spotted fevers)*: widely distributed in Africa and the Mediterranean region (boutonneuse fever), in Asia (Siberian tick typhus), Australia (Queensland tick typhus) and North America (Rocky Mountain spotted fever). Occurs in persons exposed to ticks infected from animals, such as dogs and rodents.

● *Mite-borne (scrub typhus)*: restricted to localized areas of Asia, Australia and the Pacific Islands, where suitable conditions exist for the vector mite and its rodent hosts. The disease is most common in adults occupationally exposed in forests and scrubland.

Source

● *Louse-borne*: human cases of acute typhus or recrudescent typhus (Brill–Zinsser disease); in southern USA the flying squirrel has been implicated.

● *Flea-borne*: symptomless infection in rats.

● *Tick-borne*: dogs, rabbits, rodents; may be maintained by vertical transmission in ticks.

● *Mite-borne*: field rodents.

Epidemiology

Spread

Direct person-to-person spread does not occur in typhus.

- *Louse-borne*: principally body louse, usually by scratching the site of louse bite; occasionally by inhalation of dust containing rickettsiae.
- *Flea-borne*: implantation of faeces of infected rat flea into the skin; possibly by contamination of food by infected rat's urine.
- *Tick-borne*: bite of infected tick.
- *Mite-borne*: bite of infected mite.

Pathogenesis

- In general, similar in each disease.
- Skin penetration leads rapidly to bloodstream invasion: rickettsiae penetrate endothelial cells of small vessels; endothelial damage leads to perivascular inflammation, thrombosis and vascular occlusion with tissue necrosis.
- Lipopolysaccharide endotoxin contributes to pathogenesis.
- Severe haemorrhagic manifestations due to disseminated intravascular coagulation (DIC).
- Encrusted ulcer at site of arthropod bite, may progress to eschar-formation with black, necrotic centre.
- Brill–Zinsser disease recrudescent form of epidemic typhus; rickettsiae sequestered from primary infection reactivated.

Clinical features — epidemic louse-borne typhus

Incubation period

About 1 week; extremes 4–14 days.

Onset

Sudden with chills, severe headache; myalgia and fever.

Course

Fever reaches plateau after 2 days, 39–41°C. Eyes suffused; photophobia. Rash appears on fifth day. Second week: prostrated, stuporose, deaf. Peripheral gangrene. Third week: death or recovery with fall in temperature by crisis or rapid lysis and improvement in mental state. Mortality variable, up to 60%.

Clinical features—epidemic louse-borne typhus

Rash
Appears first on upper trunk and spreads centrifugally but avoids face, palms and soles. Pinkish macules becoming maculopapular then petechial and ecchymotic. Persists for about 10 days. No eschar.

Clinical features — Brill–Zinsser disease
History of previous attack of epidemic typhus. Illness milder and of shorter duration. Rash similar but may be absent. Mortality low, 1–2%.

Clinical features — murine typhus

Incubation period
Usually 7–14 days.

Onset
Usually gradual.

Course
Similar to epidemic typhus but milder and shorter. Temperature swings more. Dry cough not uncommon. Very mild in young children. Mortality about 2%.

Rash
Present in about 70%. Appears on trunk on days 3–5 and spreads centrifugally. Macules or maculopapules. No eschar. Duration very variable.

Clinical features — tick typhus of New World (Rocky Mountain spotted fever)

Incubation period
About 7 days; may extend from 1 to 10 days.

Onset
Similar to epidemic typhus.

Clinical features—tick typhus of New World

Course
Moderately high fever persists for 10−12 days. Severe headache, myalgia and arthralgia. Rash appears about fourth day. Neurological signs common. Mortality varies with age and averages 6%.

Rash
Commences on periphery of limbs and spreads centripetally. Consists of pinkish macules becoming papular after a day or two, then petechial and ecchymotic in severe attacks. Lesions may ulcerate. Usually no eschar.

Clinical features — tick typhus of Old World
Similar to Rocky Mountain spotted fever but milder and with low mortality. Rash consists of roseolar macules or nodules and rarely becomes haemorrhagic. Tends to be profuse especially over trunk and lower limbs. Eschar frequently present and accompanied by regional lymphadenitis.

Clinical features — scrub typhus

Incubation period
Usually 6−18 days.

Course
Similar to other severe forms of typhus. Mortality variable; very low with treatment.

Rash
Appears on fifth to eighth day. Macular rash on trunk spreading to limbs. Persists for few days then fades rapidly. Eschar usually present; accompanied by lymphadenitis.

Laboratory diagnosis

Serology
• Detection of specific humoral antibodies developing during course of infection by indirect immunofluorescence, or by complement fixation; latter less sensitive.

Laboratory diagnosis

- Weil–Felix agglutination reaction utilizes antigens shared between rickettsiae and some *Proteus* spp.

Weil–Felix reaction

	Epidemic louse-borne*	Murine	Tick-borne group	Scrub
P. vulgaris OX–19	+++	+++	+	
P. vulgaris OX-2	+	+	+	
P. mirabilis OX-K			+	+++**

*Negative in Brill–Zinsser disease.
**Fifty per cent of cases.

Microscopy
Rickettsiae demonstrable by immunofluorescence in biopsy of skin lesion.

Treatment
Tetracycline 25 mg/kg daily or chloramphenicol 50 mg/kg daily for 7–14 days.

Prevention

Immediate
- Isolation: unnecessary, except in louse-borne typhus until infestation treated.
- Report to health authority.
- Notifiable in UK. Report louse-borne typhus to WHO.
- Early specific treatment.
- Delousing with malathion, lindane or DDT.
- Inspection and, if necessary, delousing of contacts. Mass delousing in epidemics.
- Rat control in murine typhus.
- Chemoprophylaxis with chloramphenicol (3 g weekly for 4 weeks) has been suggested for persons at serious risk of scrub typhus. Doxycycline may be a suitable alternative.

Prevention

Longterm
- Improve housing and social conditions.
- Control of louse infestations. Rodent control.
- Avoid tick-infested areas; wear protective clothing; use insect repellent.
- Immunization against louse-borne typhus (p. 361).

Urinary tract infections

Organisms
Enterobacteria responsible for >90% of acute infections: *Escherichia coli* cause 65–80% of total; faecal streptococci and types of coagulase-negative staphylococci account for the remainder. Wider range of pathogens, such as *Pseudomonas aeruginosa*, and sometimes mixed infections found in presence of neurogenic bladder or gross structural abnormalities of urinary tract. *Candida* spp. occasionally cause of cystitis in association with vaginitis, or following antibiotic treatment of long standing or recurrent infections. Rare condition of acute haemorrhagic cystitis of childhood associated with adenovirus types 2 and 11. Tuberculosis (p. 189).

Epidemiology

Distribution
Common infections worldwide; commoner in females than males; incidence increases with age. In UK account for approximately 12 per 1000 general practitioner consultations. Predisposing factors include urethral instrumentation, especially indwelling catheters, and conditions which impede the free flow of urine.

Source
Derived from faecal flora and may have originated from contaminated food or water.

Spread
Most *E. coli* infections are endogenous. Other organisms often introduced during surgical procedures.

Pathogenesis
Ascending infection; most common in women of child-bearing age, sometimes directly related to coitus; usually preceded by introital colonization; short female urethra and absence of antibacterial prostatic secretions believed to account for preponderance in women.

Any factor interfering with the normal flow of urine increases susceptibility to infection in both sexes and all ages; accounts for increased incidence in elderly men in association with prostatic hypertrophy. Renal lithiasis likewise predisposes to infection: phosphate stones particularly associated with infection by *Proteus* spp. (*Proteus* spp. produce urease which splits urea leading to increased ammonia concentration, high pH and consequent triple phosphate crystallization.)

Cystitis may extend, giving rise to acute pyelonephritis; rarely perinephric abscess. Chronic pyelonephritis can follow recurrent or long-standing bacterial infection; risk especially great in obstructive renal disease and in young children with vesico-ureteric reflux; can lead to end-stage renal failure (30% of childhood and 20% of adult renal failure follows chronic pyelonephritis).

Asymptomatic bacteriuria: symptomless 'significant' bacteriuria found in 1–2% of schoolgirls and 3–5% of adult women. Untreated, 30% of pregnant women with asymptomatic bacteriuria will progress to acute pyelonephritis later in pregnancy; treatment of bacteriuria greatly reduces this risk. No proven benefit from detecting and treating bacteriuria in non-pregnant women.

Clinical features
Urinary tract infections are extremely common and may involve the kidneys, ureters, bladder, prostate or urethra. It is often difficult on clinical assessment to be certain of the extent of the infection. The possibility of a predisposing cause should always be considered, especially in children and men.

Acute pyelonephritis
- Sudden onset of pain in loin radiating to the iliac fossa and suprapubic area. May be unilateral or bilateral.
- Marked general disturbance with fever, rigors and vomiting.
- Increased frequency of micturition, passing small amounts of scalding urine. Strangury. Severe bilateral infection may be accompanied by oliguria.
- Urine may be cloudy and have unpleasant smell.
- Tenderness and guarding in renal angle.
- In young children the general features dominate and the illness may present with fever and gastrointestinal disturbance.
- Complications: septicaemia, perinephric abscess, necrotizing papillitis in ureteric obstruction or in diabetics.

Clinical features

Chronic pyelonephritis
- May be no history of preceding acute episodes.
- Urinary symptoms may be absent.
- Listlessness, tiredness or vague ill health.
- Uraemia and hypertension.

Cystitis
- General disturbance slight.
- Increased frequency with scalding pain on micturition.
- Urine may be cloudy and have unpleasant smell.
- Suprapubic pain and tenderness.

Prostatitis
- Considerable general disturbance and local pain.
- Marked tenderness on rectal examination.

Urethritis (pp. 29, 107)
- Pain and urethral discharge.
- Scalding on micturition.
- May be component of syndrome, such as Reiter's disease.
- Urethral syndrome: frequency and dysuria in absence of organisms. Possibly not due to infection.

Laboratory diagnosis

Urine
- *Collection*:

Avoid contamination of specimen with urethral commensals.

Clean voided (CVSU) or suprapubic aspiration (SPA) specimens of urine are suitable.

Positive findings in clean-catch specimens from infants must be confirmed with an SPA.

Catheterization should not be performed solely to obtain urine for culture.

Specimens from patients with indwelling catheters are obtained by sterile 'venepuncture' of the collecting tube and *not* by disconnecting the system or by taking specimen from the bag.

Nevertheless, it is impossible by urine culture to differentiate bacterial colonization of the catheter or bladder, which is common in catheterized patients and does not normally warrant interference, from ascending infection.

- *Microscopy*: Uncentrifuged urine can reveal leucocytes and epithelial cells; bacteria are also visible if present in large numbers ($>10^5$ organisms/ml).
- *Culture*:

Semiquantitative methods, commonly using standard volume bacteriological loops, are usual in routine diagnostic laboratories. Quantitative dipslides are also suitable and have the advantage of possible inoculation at the time of specimen collection.

Interpretation of CVSUs

- *Microscopy*: pyuria may be present without significant bacteriuria and vice versa. Persistent pyuria in the absence of bacteriuria may indicate renal tuberculosis. Squamous epithelial cells indicate some contamination of the specimen, which must be taken into consideration when interpreting the culture findings.
- *Culture*: more than 10^5 organisms of a single species per ml urine in the presence of appropriate symptoms is highly likely to be of clinical significance. A similar result in the absence of symptoms requires culture of a further specimen; repeated findings indicate active infection with a 90% probability. Between 10^4 and 10^5 organisms/ml may indicate contamination and a further specimen should be submitted. However, acute urinary infection may be associated with fewer than 10^5 organisms/ml if:

    There is extreme frequency of micturition.

    There is considerable diuresis from increased fluid intake.

    There is some antibacterial substance (antibiotic or other) in the urine.

Follow-up cultures

Treated urinary tract infections should always have at least one follow-up culture after 6 weeks; this is necessary because symptomatic improvement may not indicate bacteriological cure. Specimens taken too soon after completion of treatment may be misleading and be followed by recrudescence of infection.

Laboratory diagnosis

Blood cultures
These should be taken from patients with suspected acute pyelonephritis or perinephric abscess (approximately 20% of Gram-negative
septicaemias originate in the urinary tract).

Other investigations
An acute attack of pyelonephritis in a child or man, or recurring
episodes in a woman, are indications for investigation of the urinary
tract to exclude a structural abnormality or the presence of a stone.
Investigations include:
● Clinical examination to detect prostatic hypertrophy in men or
vaginal prolapse in women.
● Ultrasound examination of urinary tract.
● Micturating cystography to exclude vesico-ureteric reflux.
● Excretion urography.
● Cystoscopy and retrograde pyelography.

Treatment

Acute infection
● Initial treatment may be necessary on 'best guess' basis. In hospital-
acquired infection, treatment should be based on known sensitivity of
the local organisms.
● Suitable drugs include: co-trimoxazole 2 tablets twice daily, trimethoprim 200 mg twice daily, or ampicillin 250 mg four times a day.
Continue treatment for 7 days then review in the light of culture
findings.

Recurrent infections
● Double micturition to ensure bladder is emptied.
● Longterm treatment with nitrofurantoin or nalidixic acid reduce
symptomatic recurrences.
● Treatment with these drugs should be monitored by urine culture
and is contraindicated in renal insufficiency.

Post-coital infection
● Single dose of suitable drug immediately following intercourse can
prevent post-coital cystitis.

Prevention

Immediate
- Isolation: usually unnecessary unless organism is highly resistant.
- Ensure sterility of catheters and surgical instruments.
- Careful aseptic techniques.

Longterm
- Surgical treatment of any obstruction in urinary tract.
- The role of surgery in the treatment of vesico-ureteric reflux is not established.

Varicella (chickenpox) and herpes zoster (shingles)

Organism
Herpesvirus varicellae/zoster: spherical DNA virus, approximately 150 nm in diameter. May be propagated in a variety of primary cultures of human and monkey tissues.

Epidemiology

Distribution
Infection worldwide, very common, usually mild childhood disease, rarely subclinical. Severe disease in neonates without maternal antibody, in adults and in immunocompromised, especially with leukaemia. Congenital malformations reported after infection in first trimester. General practitioner reports in UK suggest about 500 new cases per year per 100 000 population; no regular secular trends but peak in first half of year; about 20 deaths per year, over half in immunocompromised adults.

Herpes zoster: usually adults but may occur at any age and at same time as varicella; common in immunocompromised, including persons with symptomless HIV infection.

Source
Human: lesions in mouth and respiratory tract. Highly infectious just before and during the first few days of eruption. Skin lesions less infectious. Scabs not infectious. Period of infectivity may be prolonged in immunocompromised.

Spread
Direct contact, droplets or airborne.

Pathogenesis
Virus enters via the respiratory tract, where it replicates during the incubation period. Viraemia follows and virus is conveyed to the skin, where the typical vesicles develop in the epidermis. Virus then spreads centripetally along sensory nerve fibres to the dorsal root ganglia, where it remains latent. The latent virus may become reactivated at any time and travel centrifugally along the sensory nerves until it

reaches the skin, where it replicates giving rise to an attack of herpes zoster in the affected dermatome.

Clinical features — chickenpox

Incubation period
Usually 15–18 days: may extend from 7 to 26 days.

Prodromal period
Usually absent in children: adults may have fever, headache, sore throat and malaise for 1–2 days.

Rash
Evolves rapidly through stages of papule, vesicle and pustule to crust; cropping during first few days; centripetal distribution; occasionally haemorrhagic; acute stage settles after 5–7 days.

Immunodeficiency
These patients especially vulnerable.

Complications
Secondary sepsis due to *Strep. pyogenes* or *Staph. aureus*; viral pneumonia sometimes leading to miliary calcification: cerebellar encephalitis usually with complete recovery.

Clinical features — herpes zoster

Pain
Segmental distribution; associated with hyperaesthesia; present for 3–4 days before rash.

Rash
Unilateral segmental distribution; evolution similar to that of chickenpox but more scarring. Sparse generalized eruption follows in many patients; heavy rash may be found in immunocompromised.

Course
Very variable; exceptionally severe in immunodeficient patients.

Complications
Keratoconjunctivitis and iridocyclitis: meningitis, encephalitis, myelitis and lower motor neurone paralysis; secondary bacterial infection seldom troublesome; post-herpetic neuralgia common and distressing.

Laboratory diagnosis
- Confirmation of clinical diagnosis seldom necessary.
- Electron microscopy demonstrates presence of herpesvirus.
- Serology shows fourfold rise in complement-fixing or neutralizing antibody.
- Culture of virus or antigen detection by immunological methods.

Treatment

Varicella
- Usually a mild illness and little treatment required; analgesics and antihistamines in uncomplicated attack.
- Antiviral drugs for life-threatening varicella: acyclovir 10 mg/kg 8-hourly by slow i.v. infusion over 1 hour until satisfactory response, then by mouth (800 mg five times a day). Total course 5–7 days.
- Antibiotics for secondary infection.

Herpes zoster
- Analgesics for pain.
- Acyclovir by mouth for moderately severe attack: 800 mg five times a day for 7 days. Treatment should be started as soon as possible.
- Acyclovir i.v. as above for severe attack in immunodeficient patients; treatment should be started as soon as possible.
- Treatment of post-herpetic neuralgia unsatisfactory and usually consists of analgesics and mild tranquillizers.

Prevention

Immediate
- Isolation: patients with varicella requiring hospital care should be admitted to infectious diseases unit; patients with herpes zoster are potential risk to non-immune or immunocompromised and in hospi-

tal should be isolated with respiratory/wound precautions until lesions have crusted.

● Inform hospital control-of-infection officer.

● Identify hospital contacts: isolate susceptible patients and exclude susceptible staff from 10 days after first exposure to 21 days after last exposure.

● Zoster immunoglobulin (ZIG) should be given, preferably within 72 hours of exposure, to contacts with leukaemia, HIV infection, or who are otherwise immunodeficient or who are suffering from debilitating disease or who are pregnant. Dose:

    0−5 years: 250 mg.

    6−10 years: 500 mg.

    11−14 years: 750 mg.

    15+ years: 1 g i.m.

● Neonates (within 4 weeks after birth) exposed to maternal varicella (onset within 6 days before birth or whose mothers develop varicella after delivery) or other source: ZIG 250 mg i.m.

● Outside hospital: exclude from school or nursery until 6 days after onset of rash.

● Not reportable in most countries.

Longterm

● Serological screening and vaccination of susceptible patients at high risk with varicella virus vaccine if available.

● Screening of staff before working with high-risk patients; exclude susceptibles, or until protected with varicella virus vaccine.

Viral haemorrhagic fevers (VHF)

1 Arthropod-borne

Organisms
All are different types of arboviruses and are spread by arthropod
vectors. Togaviruses (>300 serotypes, which include alpha and
flaviviruses): 40–70 nm diameter; grow in tissue cultures; multiply
within arthropods, apparently without causing disease. Other
arboviruses transmitted from reservoirs of infection in small animals
and birds.

Epidemiology
See pp. 326–8.

Pathogenesis
Capable of causing severe disease, although symptomless infection
common in endemic areas; haemorrhagic manifestations probably
immune-complex mediated. Yellow fever virus invades liver causing
hepatitis.

Clinical features
See pp. 333–4.

Laboratory diagnosis

Serology
Demonstration of specific antibodies by complement fixation, haemagglutination inhibition or neutralization of cytopathogenic effects
in tissue culture.

Culture
Virus isolation of limited usefulness. Sucking mice, tissue culture cell
lines.

Treatment
See p. 334.

Epidemiology

Epidemiology — arthropod-borne VHF

Disease	Distribution	Source	Spread
Dengue haemorrhagic fever (p. 55) (flavivirus: dengue, types 1–4)	First recognized in Philippines in 1953, since then increasing reports of outbreaks in South East Asia, Pacific islands, India and 1980s in Cuba and other Caribbean islands. Not reported in Africa. Affects mainly indigenous children in these dengue endemic areas, often high mortality, rarely affects visitors or immigrants to these areas. May be caused by sensitization to a recent infection with another dengue virus type	Human, possibly monkeys	Bite of infected mosquito, usually *Aedes aegypti*. Direct person-to-person spread does not occur
'Dengue-like' chikungunya fever (alphavirus)	First described in an epidemic in Tanzania in 1952. Since reported elsewhere in Africa, India and South East Asia, often in association with dengue virus infection. Haemorrhagic disease reported in India and South East Asia but not in Africa	Human, possibly monkeys	Bite of infected mosquito, usually *Aedes aegypti*

	Epidemiology	Reservoir	Transmission
Rift Valley fever (bunyavirus: phlebovirus)	Occasional mild infections in sub-Saharan Africa associated with outbreaks of severe disease in domestic animals and endemic infection in wild game. Extensive epizootic in domestic animals in Egypt in 1977 with many associated human infections with severe haemorrhagic manifestations	Rodents, wild game, domestic animals	Bite of infected mosquito, *Culex pipiens* in Egyptian epidemic. Direct contact with blood of sick animals. Person-to-person spread not reported.
Yellow fever (flavivirus)	Confined to tropical areas of Africa and South America. Extensive urban epidemics in the past controlled in South America by mosquito eradication, now occurs mainly in adult males working in jungle areas. Urban outbreaks still occur in Africa	Man in urban areas. Monkeys in jungle areas	Bite of infected *Aedes aegypti* in urban areas, other species in jungle areas.
Crimean and Congo haemorrhagic fever; (bunyavirus: nairovirus)	Central Asia, Eastern Europe, Middle East and Africa. Late summer incidence in USSR mainly in farm workers. Outbreaks reported in persons handling infected animals and in health-care personnel associated with sick patients. High mortality especially in nosocomial outbreaks	Infected cattle, sheep and goats. Human cases	Bite of infective ticks of *Hyalomma* spp. Direct infection from handling infected animals and from contact with blood and tissue fluids of infected patients

Epidemiology

Epidemiology — arthropod-borne VHF (*continued*)

Disease	Distribution	Source	Spread
Kyasanur Forest disease (flavivirus)	First reported in Kyasanur Forest area of Mysore, India in 1957. Disease localized to this area, large epidemic in 1983	Small wild animals	Bite of infective ticks, *Haemaphysalis spinigera*
Omsk haemorrhagic fever (flavivirus)	Severe haemorrhagic fever outbreak reported 1945–48 in Omsk, Siberia. Sporadic cases since in rural workers and children exposed in tick infested forests	Rodents, muskrats	Bite of infective ticks, *Dermacentor pictus*
Korean haemorrhagic fever; nephropathia epidemica (Hantaan virus)	First recognized in Korean War in 1950s, virus isolated in 1977, shown to be also associated with haemorrhagic fever with renal syndrome in Scandinavia and eastern Europe. Small outbreak of four cases in 1977 reported in UK associated with laboratory rats. Cases also reported from other European countries	Field rodents and voles; laboratory rats	Unknown, possibly aerosol from rodent excreta

2 Zoonotic

Organisms
Lassa fever virus: arenavirus (RNA), 100 nm diameter; grows in monkey kidney cell lines. Argentine and Bolivian haemorrhagic fevers are also caused by arenaviruses.

Epidemiology
See p. 330.

Pathogenesis
- Cellular necrosis.
- Damage to vascular endothelium resulting in oedema, haemorrhage and hypovolaemic shock.
- Bone marrow suppression.
- Immune-complex deposition.
- Disseminated intravascular coagulation (DIC).

Clinical features
See pp. 333−4.

Laboratory diagnosis

Corneal scrapings
Demonstration of infected cells by immunofluorescence.

Culture
Virus isolation from blood or body fluids in tissue culture.

Serology
Indirect immunofluorescence; antibody titre>1/1024 or fourfold rise. Complement-fixing antibodies fail to develop in 50%.

Treatment
See p. 334.

Epidemiology — zoonotic VHF

Disease	Distribution	Source	Spread
Lassa fever (arenavirus)	First reported in Nigeria in 1969 as nosocomial infection with high fatality. Since this time further outbreaks have been reported in rural hospitals in West Africa and the infection has been shown to be endemic in localized rural areas. Laboratory infection of two cases in USA in 1970. Ten known importations into UK 1971–87, no spread of infection demonstrated	Multimammate rat, *Mastomys natalensis*. Symptomless excretion of virus in urine. Appears confined to this species in West Africa	Food or dust contaminated with infected rats' urine. Person-to-person spread by accidental inoculation of blood or tissue fluid from infected person. Airborne spread has been suggested
Argentine haemorrhagic fever (arenavirus: Junin)	First described in 1943. Annual outbreaks of severe illness in agricultural areas in autumn and winter; affects mainly males	Wild rodents, urine and saliva	Airborne by dust
Bolivian haemorrhagic fever (arenavirus: Machupo)	Recognized in 1959 in rural areas of northern Boliva. Localized annual outbreaks reported	Wild rodents, urine and saliva	Contaminated food and water, direct infection through abraded skin. Person-to-person spread has been described

3 Marburg and Ebola virus diseases

Organisms
Marburg virus (Green monkey disease): classified within Filoviridiae, an RNA virus, 665 x 100 nm, distinctive hooked shape; grows in various tissue-culture cell lines forming intracytoplasmic inclusions; pathogenic for wide range of laboratory animals. Ebola virus similar to Marburg virus but antigenically distinguishable.

Epidemiology
See p. 332.

Pathogenesis
Severe generalized infection presumably due to wide dissemination of virus in tissues; associated leucopenia with atypical lymphocytes.

Clinical features
See p. 334.

Laboratory diagnosis
- *Electronmicroscopy*: patient's serum during first day.
- *Culture*: virus best isolated by inoculation of blood into guinea pigs.
- *Serology*: antibody detection by indirect immunofluorescence
- *Autopsy*: detection of virus in samples of liver removed by needle.

Treatment
See p. 334.

Epidemiology — Marburg and Ebola virus diseases

Disease	Distribution	Source	Spread
Marburg (filovirus)	First described in 1967 in an outbreak of 31 cases in Marburg, Frankfurt and Belgrade in laboratory staff handling infected monkeys from Uganda, and in health-care staff who cared for the sick laboratory staff. Further incidents reported in Africa in 1975, 1980 and 1982	Probably a zoonosis; animal reservoir not known	Marburg and Ebola spread not fully known. Person-to-person spread by accidental inoculation of infected blood, tissue fluid in laboratories and hospitals. Spread by sexual intercourse has been reported
Ebola (filovirus)	Large outbreaks in Sudan and Zaire 1976 and 1979. One laboratory infection in UK in 1976 in a scientist who pricked his finger whilst working with material from the African outbreak	Probably a zoonosis; animal reservoir not known	

4 Clinical features of VHF

General features

In most instances the viral haemorrhagic fevers present as unexplained influenza-like illnesses with few distinguishing features. While the diagnosis may be suspected on epidemiological or clinical grounds laboratory confirmation is essential.

- Most VHFs have sudden onset with chills and high fever accompanied by headache, myalgia and arthralgia. Conjunctivitis common.
- Many have gastrointestinal disturbance with anorexia, nausea, vomiting and sometimes diarrhoea.
- Some have involvement of CNS with delirium, drowsiness ending in coma, and occasionally focal signs.
- All severe cases have tendency to bleed into skin, mucous membranes and internal organs.
- High mortality with death commonly in second week; terminal renal failure and circulatory collapse.

Special features

Dengue
See p. 55.

Chikungunya fever
Resembles dengue. Painful swollen joints. No shock.

Rift Valley fever
Incubation 2−4 days. Exudative retinitis and encephalitis common in Egyptian epidemic.

Yellow fever
Incubation 3−6 days. Great variation in severity. Mild cases improve after 4−5 days; severe cases have biphasic illness with further rise in temperature, bradycardia, severe prostration, jaundice, renal failure and haemorrhage.

Crimean haemorrhagic fever
Incubation 7−12 days. Gingivitis and halitosis prominent. Pneumonia

common but renal failure unusual. African infections usually subclinical or mild.

Korean haemorrhagic fever (Nephropathia epidemica)
Incubation 7−35 days, usually 14−21. About two-thirds have relatively mild illness; one-third have severe illness with haemorrhages,
shock, renal failure and pulmonary oedema.

Lassa fever
Incubation 7−21 days. Insidious onset with sore throat. Exudative
pharyngitis in some patients and occasionally small vesicles or small
ulcers on tonsils or palate. Lethargy or prostration out of proportion
to fever.

Argentine and Bolivian haemorrhagic fevers
Incubation 7−16 days. No distinctive features. CNS signs in severe
attacks.

Marburg and Ebola virus diseases
Incubation 2−21 days, usually 3−7. Vomiting and diarrhoea prominent. Characteristic morbilliform rash between days 3 and 8. Alteration
in mental state.

Treatment
- Symptomatic.
- Ribavirin given in first week of a severe attack of Lassa fever
reduces mortality by half.
- Convalescent serum containing a high level of neutralizing antibody has proved effective in treating Argentine haemorrhagic fever
and has also been advocated for Lassa fever and Marburg and Ebola
virus infections, but there is no conclusive evidence that it is beneficial
in these conditions.
- Peritoneal dialysis for renal failure.
- Blood transfusion, platelets and fresh frozen plasma for bleeding.

Prevention

Immediate
- Isolation: high-security isolation for Lassa fever, Marburg and Ebola virus infections, and Crimean−Congo haemorrhagic fever until virus can no longer be detected; needle and wound precautions for arbovirus infections; strict precautions for other VHF.
- Meticulous attention to prevent accidental inoculation of health-care and laboratory staff with blood or body fluids.
- Report to health authority; notifiable in UK. Report required to WHO for yellow fever.
- Inform hospital control-of-infection officer.
- Consider use of ribavirin for chemoprophylaxis of Lassa fever.
- Nurse patients in tropics or subtropics with mosquito-borne infections under mosquito nets.
- Investigate source and spread.
- In yellow fever, immunize contacts as soon as possible; vaccine gives protection in 7 days.
- Surveillance of contacts of Lassa fever, Marburg and Ebola virus diseases, and Crimean−Congo fever for 21 days; contacts defined as persons who attended the patient during the illness, or who handled the patient's blood, urine or secretions, or who had contact with the corpse of a deceased patient; record temperature daily, consider admission to hospital if temperature above 38°C for more than 24 hours.
- Contacts need not be excluded from work as long as they remain afebrile.

Longterm
- Rodent control.
- Vector control.
- High standards of hospital and laboratory practice to avoid accidental transmission, especially when caring for patients from known endemic areas.
- Yellow fever immunization (p. 362).

Yersinia infections

1 Plague

Organism
Yersinia pestis: small Gram-negative rod, previously included in the genus *Pasteurella*: in clinical material capsulated and shows bipolar staining.

Epidemiology

Distribution
Widespread zoonosis with persistent foci of infection in wild rodents in South East Asia, Indonesia, India, Africa, western USA and South America. Although urban plague has been controlled in most parts of the world, sporadic human cases continue to occur in rural areas with endemic rodent infection. The threat of infection spreading to urban rat population, resulting in epizootics followed by epidemics in the human population, remains. In the USA up to 40 cases reported per year 1980–86; in UK none since 1919 apart from a laboratory infection in 1962.

Source
Wild rodents, ground squirrels in USA, sometimes hares and rabbits, household rats.

Spread
Transmitted by bite of rat flea. Reported in persons handling tissues of infected animals and laboratory cultures. Person-to-person transmission by droplets from human cases of pneumonic plague or pets with plague pneumonia.

Pathogenesis
From site of implantation, organism spreads via the lymphatics to regional lymph nodes and thence to bloodstream. Protective capsule formed, and organism able to proliferate within mononuclear phagocytes. Lipopolysaccharide endotoxin liberated from cell wall contributes to toxaemia and haemorrhagic manifestations.

Clinical features — bubonic plague

Incubation period
Usually 3–4 days; may extend from 2 to 10 days.

Onset
Sudden with sharp rise in temperature to 40°C or higher.

Bubo
Lymph nodes draining area of infected bite become tender and swell rapidly. Inguinal in 70%: axillary in 20%. Surrounding oedema sometimes haemorrhagic. Late suppuration with discharge and secondary infection.

Mental state
Dullness and apathy progressing to stupor and prostration.

Skin
Haemorrhages into and under skin; also in mucous membranes. Ischaemic necrosis produces black patches (Black Death).

Course
From 30 to 90% die about fifth day. Septicaemia leading to circulatory failure; DIC common. Secondary plague pneumonia in later stages. Occasionally septic meningitis. Often epigastric pain, nausea, vomiting and sometimes diarrhoea.

Clinical features — pneumonic plague

Incubation period
Usually 2–3 days.

Onset
Abrupt rise in temperature. Severe malaise. Signs of pneumonia appear on second day. Frequent cough with mucoid, watery sputum later becoming bloodstained.

Clinical features—pneumonic plague

Course
Severe pain in chest and rapidly increasing respiratory distress.
Septicaemia invariable. Profuse haemorrhages. Circulatory failure
and death after 2–3 days.

Laboratory diagnosis

Microscopy
Organisms usually numerous; can be demonstrated by Gram,
methylene blue or immunofluorescent staining of fluid from vesicle
at site of entry, lymph node aspirate, or sputum in pulmonary
infection.

Culture
Isolation from blood culture, or from pus and sputum. Grows on
simple media, optimally at 30°C; differentiated from other *Yersinia*
spp. and pasteurellae by biochemical tests and with specific antisera.

Serology
Specific antibodies are produced during the course of the disease.

Treatment — bubonic plague
- Tetracycline, streptomycin or sulphonamides.

Treatment — meningitis
- Chloramphenicol.

Treatment — pneumonic plague
- Tetracycline or streptomycin systemically.

Prevention

Immediate
- Isolation: strict precautions in pneumonic plague; wound pre-
cautions in bubonic plague.
- Early specific treatment.
- Disinfestation.

Prevention

- Report to health authority; notifiable in UK. Report required to WHO.
- Identify household and other close contacts; surveillance for 7 days; chemoprophylaxis with tetracycline 500 mg four times a day for 7 days, or sulphadimidine or sulphadiazine 2−4 g daily for 7 days.

Longterm
- Rodent and flea control
- Immunization (p. 360).

2 Other infections

Organisms
Yersinia enterocolitica and *Y. pseudotuberculosis* (several sero-types): two closely related species of small Gram-negative rods; previously included in the genus *Pasteurella*.

Epidemiology

Distribution
Worldwide zoonoses affecting many species of wild and domestic animals and birds. Uncommon sporadic infection apparently increasing in Europe and North America; outbreaks reported in schools; community outbreaks associated with contaminated food also reported.

Source
Domestic food animals, particularly pigs, and pets.

Spread
Faecal−oral spread from animals, and from person to person. Foodborne and milkborne infections reported.

Pathogenesis
Ill understood. Presumably infection contracted via the gastro-intestinal tract extends to regional lymphatics; bacteraemia believed to occur occasionally. It is suggested that hepatic dysfunction or dis-

ordered iron metabolism is responsible for rare septicaemic infections with *Y. pseudotuberculosis*, possibly also with *Y. enterocolitica*.

Clinical features

Incubation
3–7 days.

Y. enterocolitica
● Enterocolitis: mainly in young children; fever, diarrhoea and abdominal pain.
● Acute ileitis and mesenteric lymphadenitis: older children and adults; similar in presentation to acute appendicitis.
● Arthritis: affects up to one-third of adults within 2 weeks of acute attack of enterocolitis; HLA-B27 antigen present in 90%; joints of lower limbs most severely involved; erythema nodosum common.
● Septicaemia: rare, mainly in elderly; fever, abdominal pain and visceral abscess formation; high mortality.

Y. pseudotuberculosis
● Presents clinically as acute appendicitis; appendix normal; mesenteric lymph nodes swollen and inflamed.
● Occasionally erythema nodosum and polyarthritis.
● Septicaemia very rare.

Laboratory diagnosis

Culture
● Isolation from mesenteric lymph nodes at laparotomy or from blood culture in septicaemic cases is straightforward.
● Faecal cultures positive in acute stage of illness but laboratory should be alerted so that the relatively insignificant colonies are not overlooked.
● Identification by biochemical reactions, confirmed by agglutination with specific antisera.

Laboratory diagnosis

Serology
A rising titre of specific antibodies demonstrable during course of the illness.

Treatment
- Infection usually self-limiting.
- Antibiotic therapy indicated for septicaemia but choice uncertain and response poor. Possibly gentamicin or chloramphenicol for *Y. enterocolitica* and ampicillin, tetracycline or gentamicin for *Y. pseudotuberculosis*
- Arthritis does not respond to antibiotics. Aspirin or non-steroidal anti-inflammatory drug for symptomatic relief.

Prevention

Immediate
- Isolation: enteric precautions.
- Report to health authority.
- Search for possible associated cases by reviewing cases of enteritis and appendicitis to identify outbreaks.
- Investigation and control of source.

Longterm
- Personal and food hygiene to prevent faecal–oral and foodborne spread.
- Pasteurization of milk.

Appendix A: Chemoprophylaxis

Widespread use of prophylactic antibiotics is potentially dangerous. Risks include:

- Eradication of normally sensitive commensal flora and its replacement with more antibiotic-resistant organisms; the latter may give rise to infection which presents therapeutic problems.
- Induction of antibiotic resistance in microorganisms, including commensal species; resistance may be transferable to pathogenic species and may extend to include other unrelated drugs.
- Development of hypersensitivity, precluding subsequent use in therapy.

Chemoprophylaxis must not be used at the expense of other methods of reducing infection, e.g. avoidance of contact, or maintenance of high standards of asepsis and surgical technique.

Antibiotic prophylaxis is valuable where the risk of severe infection is clearly defined and when it cannot be reduced or eliminated by other means.

- Drugs selected should be appropriate against the recognized pathogens and of as narrow a spectrum as possible.
- Time and duration of administration must be carefully tailored to the risk.
- Route of administration must be appropriate.
- Protocols should be revised regularly with reference to altered patterns of sensitivity or changing need.
- New indications or regimens should not be introduced without proper trials.

Some indications for prophylaxis are generally accepted; others are more controversial; yet others have not been adequately assessed.

Appendix A: Chemoprophylaxis

Uses for chemoprophylaxis

Condition	Indication	Organism	Antibiotics	Duration
Rheumatic fever	To prevent subsequent attacks	*Strep. pyogenes* (all serotypes)	Benzathine penicillin, phenoxymethyl-penicillin or sulphadimidine	Children: until 20 years Adults: for 5 years after illness (see p. 282)
Endocarditis	To prevent bacter-aemia becoming estab-lished in patients with underlying heart lesion			
	• Dentistry	Viridans streptococci	Amoxycillin (orally), *or* Benzylpenicillin and gentamicin (i.m.)	1 hour before At induction of anaesthesia: for <24 hours depending on extent of procedure
	⊛ Termination of pregnancy, normal childbirth, insertion of IUCD, urogenital or gastrointestinal tract instrumentation	Faecal streptococci	Amoxycillin (orally, and gentamicin (i.m.)	1 hour before
	• Open cardiac surgery	*Staph. aureus, Staph. epidermidis,* diphtheroids	Benzylpenicillin, flucloxacillin and gentamicin (i.v.)	Immediately pre-operatively: for 48 hours; repeat with any further procedures, e.g. removal of drainage tubes

Uses for chemoprophylaxis

Uses for chemoprophylaxis (*continued*)

Condition	Indication	Organism	Antibiotics	Duration
Meningitis	For close contacts	*N. meningitidis*	Sulphadiazine, if strain sensitive; rifampicin if resistant	See p. 185
		H. influenzae	Rifampicin	See pp. 114, 185
	Recurrent infection following head injury	*Strep. pneumoniae*	Phenoxymethyl-penicillin	Longterm
After splenectomy	To reduce risk of pneumococcal infection	*Strep. pneumoniae*	Phenoxymethyl-penicillin	Possibly throughout early childhood
Recurrent urinary infection	• Children with vesicoureteric reflux	Enterobacteria	Nitrofurantoin, trimethoprim, or nalidixic acid	• Until reflux resolves or is corrected
	• After sexual intercourse			• Single dose related to risk
Prophylaxis of pyelonephritis of pregnancy by treatment of silent bacteriuria of pregnancy		Enterobacteria commonly *E. coli*	As indicated by sensitivity testing	7–10 days
Cholera	Family contacts	*V. cholerae*	Tetracycline	5–7 days (see p. 37)
Diphtheria	Unimmunized, close contacts	*C. diphtheriae*	Erythromycin or penicillin	5 days; also immunization (see p. 60)
Tetanus	After injury, depending upon risk	*Cl. tetani*	Parenteral penicillin or erythromycin, or metronidazole	Commence before wound toilet—5 days; also immunization (see p. 292)

Uses for chemoprophylaxis

Leprosy	Child household contact	*M. leprae*	Dapsone	3 years (see p. 201)
Listeriosis	Newborn infants of infected mothers	*L. monocytogenes*	Ampicillin	Not evaluated; 2–3 days
Mothers and neonates: group B streptococcal infection	Bacteriologically positive mothers and neonates; at-risk infants (e.g. premature or after prolonged membrane rupture)	Group B streptococci	Penicillin to mother and/or neonate	Not evaluated; 2–3 days
Anthrax	Persons heavily exposed	*B. anthracis*	Penicillin	1 day (p. 9)
Scrub typhus	Those at special risk	*R. tsutsugamushi*	Chloramphenicol or doxycycline	4 weeks (see p. 313)
Malaria	Travel to or through malarial zones	*Plasmodium* spp. especially *P. falciparum*	Proguanil, pyrimethamine, or chloroquine	As indicated for drug, including post-exposure (see p. 168)
Influenza	At-risk contacts in institutional outbreaks of influenza A	Influenza A virus	Amantadine	10–14 days (see p. 145)
Herpes simplex	• Immunodeficiency • Recurring attacks	Herpes simplex virus	Acyclovir	• Indefinitely (p. 132) • Interrupted every 6–12 months (p. 131)

Appendix B: Infection control

Control of infectious disease in the UK is a local responsibility, coordinated and supported by the CDSC and CD(S)U. It is the legal duty of the clinician to notify the local medical officer for environmental health (MOEH) in England and Wales and the chief administrative medical officer (CAMO) in Scotland if he or she becomes aware or suspects that a patient is suffering from any of the notifiable diseases listed in the table below. The objectives of notification are to enable rapid preventive action to be taken when appropriate, for local and national surveillance of disease and for legal purposes such as exclusion from work.

Although non-notifiable diseases are not defined it is the responsibility of the MOEH, CAMO and other community physicians to detect and measure disease in their district and to initiate preventive action.

Responsibility for control of infection in hospitals is delegated to the control-of-infection officer, usually a microbiologist, supported by an infection control nurse; both are normally members of a district control-of-infection committee and work closely together to monitor and take action to prevent hospital infection.

Notifiable infectious diseases, England and Wales 1988

Acute encephalitis	Measles	Rubella
Acute poliomyelitis	Meningitis	Scarlet fever
Anthrax	Meningococcal	Smallpox
Cholera	septicaemia	Tetanus
Diphtheria	Mumps	Tuberculosis
Dysentery, amoebic	Ophthalmia	Typhoid fever
and bacillary	neonatorum	Typhus fever
Food poisoning	Paratyphoid fever	Viral haemorrhagic
Leprosy	Plague	fever
Leptospirosis	Rabies	Viral hepatitis
Malaria	Relapsing fever	Whooping cough
		Yellow fever

Importance of infection control in hospital

Surveys in the UK and other western countries reveal that approximately 20% of inpatients have infections, half acquired prior to admission and half hospital-acquired (nosocomial infection). Factors

contributing to the acquisition and spread of nosocomial infections include:
- Close proximity of other patients.
- Surgical operations and other invasive procedures, which breach the skin or mucosal defences.
- Underlying organic disease which may predispose to infection.
- Extremes of age.
- Use of antibiotics, which encourage the emergence and persistence of antibiotic-resistant organisms in the hospital environment and interfere with the commensal flora of individuals, permitting colonization and then infection with resistant strains.
- Immunodeficiency.

Thus opportunities for infection are greater within hospital than elsewhere and therefore action is taken to control the following:
- Recognized infectious diseases.
- Undiagnosed but potentially transmissible infections.
- Certain infections in patients and staff, which outside hospital would not require special measures.
- Patient or staff carriers of certain micro-organisms.

Identification of sources of infection, (e.g. other patients, staff, visitors, food and the environment) and knowledge of routes of transmission (e.g. person-to-person contact or via inanimate objects, droplet inhalation, injection and ingestion) are necessary before effective control measures can be instituted.

General methods

Handwashing
The hands of clinical staff are the chief vehicles for spread of infection and therefore handwashing between each patient contact is the single most important method of reducing transmission. Hands should be washed thoroughly under running water using soap, or as an additional precaution an antibacterial cleanser or alcohol-based antibacterial hand rub.

Other methods of general application
- Non-touch techniques for managing wounds and carrying out all invasive procedures.
- Sterilization of all invasively-used clinical instruments by heat treatment whenever possible.
- Safe disposal of all contaminated dressings and instruments.
- Heat treatment, whenever possible, of all bedpans and urinals after use.
- High standards of hygiene in food preparation, domestic cleaning and laundry.

Specific methods

Containment (source) isolation
This is used to protect other patients and staff from an infectious patient and may be practised at different levels of security.
- *Side room of general ward*: usually an inadequate facility because staff are likely to be in common between ward and side room, discipline and hygienic practices may not be as rigorous as in a dedicated isolation facility, and it is impossible to control airborne spread unless specially ventilated.
- *Isolation ward*: provides isolation facility in single rooms, ideally with air-locks and low air-pressure relative to central parts of ward and staffed by designated specially trained nurses.
- *Infectious diseases department*: specialized unit for admission of community or hospital-acquired infection; purpose-built with safe access, single isolation rooms, designated specialist staff, controlled ventilation and special facilities for sterilization and for safe disposal of waste: limited access; special immunization and surveillance of personnel.
- *High-security isolation unit*: specialized unit, usually attached to an infectious diseases department, for secure management of patients with diseases considered to be dangerous or highly infectious.

Protective (reverse) isolation
Used for protection of patients at increased risk of acquiring infection, e.g. immunocompromised, extensive non-infected burns and certain skin diseases. Facilities likely to include: single rooms with filtered air

supply at positive-pressure relative to central ward area; sterile protective clothing for personnel entering the room; disinfection of all objects in patient's environment; sterile food.

Categories of containment isolation

Two philosophies have been accepted for containment isolation:
- An overall policy of simple barrier isolation practised to a high standard and applied to most patients with special measures taken for certain patients, e.g. those suspected of having a viral haemorrhagic fever.
- A qualified policy of barrier isolation designed to prevent transmission of a particular disease by blocking the known route of transmission.

Both methods are satisfactory when practised efficiently. The second method, which has been accepted in many hospitals, classifies the precautions to be taken according to the route of spread. The appropriate category of isolation is decided on admission or when infection is suspected and may be changed if the patient's clinical condition alters, e.g. a post operative HBsAg-positive patient should be nursed with wound and needle precautions until the operation wound has healed, when needle precautions only are necessary. The following categories are in use.

Needle precautions
- Applicable during venepuncture or similar invasive procedure.
- Avoidance of 'sharps' injury.
- Safe disposal of needles and other 'sharps'.
- Precautions, as stipulated locally, for submission of laboratory specimens.
- Single room unnecessary.

Wound precautions
- Use of single room, whenever possible, for isolation.
- Careful aseptic techniques for wound dressings.
- Staff wear gloves and gowns or disposable aprons for all patient contact.
- Safe disposal of all dressings, discharges and secretions.

Categories of containment isolation

Enteric precautions
- Single room or ward designated for patients with same disease.
- Facilities for safe disposal of all excreta and for disinfection of bedpans and urinals after use. Designated toilets.
- Disposal of apron or change of gown after dealing with infected material.
- Treatment or safe disposal of eating utensils and contaminated linen and other items.
- Visiting restricted.

Respiratory precautions
- Single room, preferably under negative-pressure and with anteroom.
- All personnel entering room to wear high-efficiency mask and disposable gloves, when dealing with more dangerous infections, and a gown or disposable apron.
- Safe disposal of nasopharyngeal secretions and sputum.
- Treatment or safe disposal of contaminated linen and other items.
- Visiting restricted.

Strict isolation
- Single room with negative-pressure filtered ventilation and anteroom.
- All personnel entering room wear impermeable gown, gloves, cap and high-efficiency mask; goggles or visor and protective footwear should be available.
- Safe disposal of excreta, discharges and blood.
- Treatment and safe disposal of eating utensils, sheets, pillow cases and other items used by the patient.
- Special care when collecting and transporting specimens to laboratory.
- Staff under surveillance if deemed necessary.
- Visiting prohibited.
- Terminal disinfection.

High-security isolation
- Purpose-built separate self-contained unit with safe access;

negative-pressure filtered ventilation; special facilities for safe auto-claving and incineration of waste.

- Specially trained staff; changing and showering facilities for staff; access restricted to approved personnel and daily surveillance of personnel.
- Use of flexible-film negative-pressure patient isolators or full protective clothing and respirators.
- Designated high-security laboratory for diagnostic and patient management tests.

Appendix C: Immunization

Active immunization

Active immunity may be acquired naturally following infection or induced artificially by administering vaccines. Develops slowly but usually lifelong duration. Live vaccines are prepared by attenuation of organisms, decreasing their virulence but retaining their ability to induce immunity, and a single dose usually confers longterm immunity, (e.g. measles and rubella). Inactivated vaccines are prepared from killed whole organisms, non-infectious subunits of organisms, or toxins, so that they are non-pathogenic but retain the ability to stimulate immune response; several doses of some vaccines are required at appropriate intervals to produce durable immunity (e.g. diphtheria and pertussis), whilst other vaccines require only a single dose (e.g. meningococcal and pneumococcal vaccines).

Storage of vaccines

Most vaccines gradually lose potency, some rapidly at high temperatures (e.g. oral poliovaccine), and must be stored carefully according to instructions on the package.

- Store at rear of well-maintained refrigerator at about +4°C.
- Do not freeze inactivated vaccines.
- Live vaccine may be frozen but must be used immediately after reconstitution.
- Do not expose vaccines to sunlight or to heat.
- Discard partly used multidose containers at end of session.

Administration of vaccines

The main principles are:

- Parental consent is required for childhood immunization.
- Immunization procedures should either be carried out by a doctor or supervised by a doctor on the premises. The responsibility may be delegated to a nurse, provided that the nurse has been trained and is competent in all aspects of immunization including anaphylaxis.
- Anaphylactic reactions are very rare but may be fatal. They manifest with pallor, apnoea, swelling of the mouth and throat, hoarseness or stridor, hypotension or urticarial rash. Adrenaline injection 1 : 1000 (1 mg/ml) and hydrocortisone should always be available for use if this emergency should arise. Dose of adrenaline i.m.: <1 year 0.05 ml: 1 year 0.1 ml: 2 years 0.2 ml: 3−4 years 0.3 ml;

5 years 0.4 ml: 6–10 years 0.5 ml; >10 years 0.5–1 ml, repeated to a maximum of three doses if necessary. Hydrocortisone 25–100 mg i.v. and repeated if necessary.

- Check manufacturer's instructions, the identity of the vaccine and expiry date.
- Always record details of the vaccine, including batch number, in the vaccinee's record.
- Oral poliovaccine may be given in syrup or directly into the mouth of young infants and on a sugar lump to older children and adults.
- Injected vaccines should normally be given into the upper arm, deep subcutaneously or i.m. into the deltoid using a 23-gauge needle; in very small babies the anterolateral thigh is recommended; intra-dermal injections should be given into the skin over the insertion of the deltoid using a 25-gauge needle.
- Jet injectors should not be used because they may transmit infections, such as hepatitis B, and are not consistently reliable.
- Prepare skin by cleaning with antiseptic, such as isopropyl alcohol, and allow to dry.
- Inactivated vaccines may be given at the same time in combined preparations or in single preparations into separate sites.
- An interval of 3 weeks is usually recommended between the administration of any two live vaccines.
- Live vaccines, except yellow fever vaccine, should not be given within 3 weeks before and 3 months after the administration of immunoglobulin.

General contraindications to immunization

- Acute illness: postpone immunization. Minor infections without fever are not a contraindication.
- Severe febrile reaction or neurological symptoms following immunization are a contraindication to further doses of the same antigen or antigens, especially pertussis.
- Live vaccines should not be given to patients with immunode-ficiency or immunosuppression.
- During pregnancy, live vaccines, (e.g. polio or yellow fever) should not normally be given, and measles and rubella vaccination should always be postponed. Similarly, immunization with inactivated vaccines should be delayed whenever possible.

General contraindications to immunization

- HIV antibody-positive individuals, with or without symptoms, should be given appropriate live and killed vaccines but not BCG or yellow fever vaccine (p. 139).
- Vaccines prepared in chick embryo, (e.g. measles, mumps, influenza or yellow fever) should not be given to persons with a history of anaphylaxis after consuming hens' eggs.
- Some vaccines contain traces of antibiotics, e.g. oral poliovaccine. Manufacturers should be consulted before administration to persons with extreme antibiotic sensitivity.
- Asthma, eczema, hay fever, prematurity, above age given in schedule, and stable neurological conditions are *not* contraindications to immunization.

Side effects of immunization

Local pain and swelling at the site of injection may occur after inactivated bacterial vaccines (e.g. pertussis or typhoid) and after repeated doses of toxoids (e.g. tetanus). Persistent suppuration may follow BCG vaccination, especially if the injection is inadvertently given subcutaneously instead of intradermally. Mild general side-effects sometimes follow vaccination, such as rash and fever about 7 days after measles vaccination, mild arthralgia following rubella vaccination and swelling of the face in the third week after mumps vaccination, but severe side effects are very rare.

- Report severe side-effects to health authority. In UK also inform Committee on Safety of Medicines (CSM); report forms available from the British National Formulary *or* from CSM, 1 Nine Elms Lane, London SW8 5NQ (tel. 01-720 2188).
- Measles vaccine (live-attenuated): encephalitis about one in 100 000 vaccinees.
- Pertussis vaccine: febrile convulsions may follow immunization, but there is no evidence that pertussis immunization causes permanent neurological damage.
- Poliovaccine (live-attenuated): association between vaccination and paralysis in about one in 2 million vaccinees, and in close contacts of about one in 2 million vaccinated. Some of these paralytic illnesses may be vaccine-induced.

Childhood immunization

In the UK routine immunization in childhood is offered against diphtheria, tetanus, pertussis, poliomyelitis, measles, mumps, rubella and tuberculosis. In the USA *Haemophilus influenzae* type b polysaccharide vaccine is also offered and BCG is not normally given. A suggested schedule adapted from the recommendations of the UK Departments of Health is given below; the vaccines are normally available free of charge from health authorities.

Approximate age	Vaccines	Comments
3 months	Diphtheria/tetanus/pertussis adsorbed (DT/Per/Vac/Ads) + oral poliovaccine (OPV)	May be given at monthly intervals if pertussis prevalent, or course begun late
5 months	DT/Per/Vac/Ads + OPV	If course interrupted it should be resumed but not repeated
10 months	DT/Per/Vac/Ads + OPV	
12–24 months	Measles/mumps/rubella (MMR)	May be given at any age over 12 months
5 years (school entry)	DT/Vac/Ads + OPV + MMR if not previously given	These three vaccines may be given at the same time
10–14 years	BCG	Give only to children who are tuberculin-negative or weakly positive
10–14 years (girls)	Rubella if not previously vaccinated with MMR	
15–19 years (school leaving)	OPV + Tet/Vac/Ads	May be given earlier, at same time as BCG

Pertussis (p. 209)
- Vaccine: killed whole-cell vaccine prepared from organisms of commonly occurring serotypes containing the three main *Bordetella*

pertussis agglutinogens; acellular vaccines have been used in Japan, field trials of efficacy are planned in UK; usually administered as a combined vaccine with diphtheria and tetanus toxoids (triple antigen); adsorbed vaccines (usually aluminium hydroxide) are preferred because they are more immunogenic and give rise to fewer local and systemic reactions.

- Dose: three doses 0.5 ml by deep subcutaneous or i.m. injection.
- Recommendations: begin at age 3 months (see schedule p. 355), reinforcing doses may be given at age 4–6 years especially if unimmunized younger siblings in the household, not recommended over 6 years of age.
- Contraindications: previously severe reaction to pertussis vaccine. Stable neurological conditions, a history of cerebral damage in neonatal period, or of convulsions, or of idiopathic epilepsy in parents or siblings are not now considered contraindications. When pertussis immunization is contraindicated immunization with diphtheria and tetanus toxoids alone should be considered.

Diphtheria (p. 57)
- Vaccine: cell-free preparation of diphtheria toxin treated with formalin; usually given to children as 'triple' adsorbed vaccine (see schedule p. 355); low-dose preparation of diphtheria toxoid available for persons over 10 years.
- Dose: primary course of three doses 0.5 ml with reinforcing dose 0.5 ml, deep subcutaneous or i.m. injection.
- Recommendations: begin at age 3 months (see schedule p. 355), reinforcing dose at school entry or at least 3 years after completion of primary course. Previously unimmunized children — three doses at monthly intervals with later reinforcing dose.
- Immunization of adults likely to be exposed to infection in hospitals: primary immunization Dip/Vac/Ads for adults — 0.5 ml i.m. three doses at monthly intervals, or single reinforcing dose. If immunization history is not known Schick test may be performed: positive = non-immune and primary immunization required; negative = immune and reinforcing dose only.
- Contraindications: see general contraindications (p. 355); use only low-dose preparations of toxoid for persons over 10 years of age.

Childhood immunization

Tetanus (p. 290)

● Vaccine: cell-free preparation of tetanus toxin treated with formalin; usually given to children as 'triple' adsorbed vaccine or combined with diphtheria toxoid or alone (see schedule p. 355).

● Dose: as diphtheria toxoid (see p. 355).

● Recommendations: begin at age 3 months (see schedule p. 355), reinforcing doses at school entry or at least 3 years after completion of primary course, and at school leaving about 10 years later; subsequent reinforcing doses in the absence of injury probably unnecessary. Previously unimmunized children and adults should be given full primary immunization, two doses at an interval of 6–12 weeks and a third dose 4–12 months later.

● Contraindications: see general contraindications (p. 355); reinforcing doses at less than 5-year intervals should not be given to the injured because they may give rise to hypersensitivity.

Poliomyelitis (p. 77)

● Vaccines: oral poliovaccine (OPV), polioviruses 1, 2 and 3 attenuated by passage in monkey-kidney cells; inactivated poliovaccine (IPV), polioviruses types 1, 2 and 3 cultured in monkey-kidney cells and inactivated with formalin.

● Dose: OPV — primary course of three doses of three drops orally with reinforcing dose; IPV — primary course of three doses, 0.5 ml deep subcutaneous or i.m. injection with reinforcing dose.

● Recommendations: OPV — begin at 3 months (see schedule p. 355), should not be given at less than 4-week intervals, reinforcing dose on school entry and leaving, and again at 10-year intervals if likely to be exposed to infection in endemic areas or in health-care workers; IPV — should be used instead of OPV in immunocompromised persons and their household members.

● Contraindications: see general contraindications (p. 355); diarrhoea or vomiting may prevent effective immunization with OPV; both OPV and IPV should not be given to persons with extreme sensitivity to antibiotics (consult vaccine manufacturer).

Measles (p. 170)

● Vaccine: freeze-dried live-attenuated vaccine, available also in combination with mumps and rubella vaccines (MMR).

- Dose: single dose, 0.5 ml deep subcutaneous or i.m. injection.
- Recommendations: age 1–2 years (see schedule p. 355); efficacy reduced under 1 year because of maternal antibody; MMR may be given at any age over 1 year and at the same time as reinforcing doses of OPV and DT/Ads vaccine.
- Contraindications: see general contraindications (p. 355); measles vaccination may temporarily inhibit response to tuberculin, and therefore tuberculin tests should be postponed for 4 weeks after vaccination; measles vaccine should not be given to persons with severe allergy to hens' eggs.

Rubella (p. 241)
- Vaccine: freeze-dried live-attenuated vaccine (Wistar RA 27/3) grown in human diploid cell cultures, available also as MMR.
- Dose: single dose, 0.5 ml subcutaneous injection.
- Recommendations: MMR aged 1–2 years (see schedule p. 355) or at school entry if not previously vaccinated; rubella vaccine in non-pregnant, seronegative women of childbearing age — who should be advised against pregnancy within 1 month of vaccination; pregnant women found to be seronegative should be vaccinated after delivery; seronegative health-service staff of both sexes, particularly those working in antenatal clinics.
- Contraindications: see general contraindications (p. 355). Immunization is contraindicated during pregnancy because vaccine virus may infect the fetus, although no malformations have been reported. For inadvertent immunization during pregnancy, termination may be considered.

Mumps (p. 186)
- Vaccine: live-attenuated vaccine available in combination with measles and rubella (MMR). See measles (p. 357) and rubella above.

Tuberculosis (p. 189)
- Vaccine: freeze-dried live-attenuated vaccine derived from *Mycobacterium bovis*; preparations for intradermal injection and for multiple puncture application are available which are *not* interchangeable. Jet injectors should not be used.
- Dose: single dose, 0.1 ml (0.05 ml in infants) intradermally, over

insertion of deltoid muscle; in all subjects except infants vaccination should be preceded by a tuberculin test.

● Recommendations: BCG vaccination should be considered in six groups of persons:

School children (see schedule p. 355); in special circumstances it may be given routinely at an earlier age, e.g. at birth.

Students, including those at teacher training colleges.

Children and newborn infants in families of Asian origin because of high incidence of tuberculosis in this ethnic group.

Health-care workers and others likely to be exposed to infection at work.

Household contacts of persons known to be suffering from active tuberculosis and newborn infants in households where there is a history of tuberculosis.

Children and young adults who are travelling to, or will reside in, areas where there is a high risk of infection.

It is usually unnecessary to revaccinate persons who have a recognizable BCG scar of at least 4 mm in diameter.

● Contraindications: see general contraindications (p. 355); persons who are immunocompromised, including those with HIV infection, should not be given BCG vaccine.

Immunization for travel

An international certificate of vaccination against yellow fever is required by some countries; a medical certificate of immunization against cholera may also be required. Other immunizations such as poliomyelitis and typhoid, although not compulsory, are desirable; malarial prophylaxis is essential for many countries (p. 168). See *Vaccination Requirements for International Travel and Health Advice to Travellers* (WHO), and in UK DHSS booklets SA40 and SA41, *The Travellers' Guide to Health*. Advice by telephone is available from: DHSS, London (tel. 01−407 5522); Medical Advisory Service for Travellers Abroad (MASTA), London (tel. 01−631 4408); Communicable Disease Surveillance Centre, London (tel. 01−200 6868); London School of Hygiene and Tropical Medicine (tel. 01−636 8636 ext 212); recorded message on malarial prophylaxis (tel. 01−636 7921); Department of Communicable and Tropical Diseases, Birmingham (tel. 021−772 4311); Liverpool School of Tropical Medicine (tel. 051−708

9393); Communicable Diseases, (Scotland) Unit, Glasgow (tel. 041–946 7120); British Airways Immunization Centres, London, also provide immunization clinics (tel. 01–439 9584, 606 2977, 562 5825).

Cholera (p. 35)
- Vaccine: heat-killed, phenol-preserved, whole-cell vaccine.
- Dose: primary immunization two doses 0.5 ml then 1.0 ml, deep subcutaneous or i.m. injection 2–3 weeks apart (smaller doses for children — see manufacturers' instructions); reinforcing dose every 6 months under epidemic conditions. Vaccine efficacy very low, only about 50% protection.
- Recommendations: travellers to countries where cholera is present, especially in areas of poor sanitation. International certificates no longer required but some countries still demand medical certificate of vaccination — valid 6 days after first injection or from reinforcing dose, for 6 months.
- Contraindications: previous severe reaction to cholera vaccine. Not recommended during pregnancy or for children under 1 year of age.

Japanese B encephalitis (p. 70)
Inactivated vaccines recommended for persons likely to be under continuous exposure in China, Japan, Korea and other countries in Asia where locally prepared vaccines are available. Japanese vaccine is available in UK for named persons, not necessarily effective outside Japan.

Meningococcal meningitis (p. 182)
Polysaccharide vaccine, monovalent group C, bivalent groups A and C, quadrivalent groups A, C, Y and W-135. Recommended in single dose over 2 years of age in outbreaks due to these types in closed or semiclosed communities and for residents in areas of high incidence and travellers to these areas. Under 2 years, two doses 3 months apart are necessary to give protection.

Plague (p. 336)
Formalin-killed, phenol-preserved vaccine. Primary course of two doses at about 4-week intervals, reinforcing doses 3–6 months later, thereafter at 6–12 months if continuing exposure. Recommended for

persons who will have frequent contact with rodents in enzootic areas and for laboratory workers handling the organism.

Poliomyelitis (p. 77)
Recommended for travellers to endemic areas, see childhood immunization (p. 357).

Typhus (p. 309)
Inactivated and live vaccines have been prepared. Recommended for persons in endemic areas and travellers to these areas. Vaccines not commercially available in North America or UK; may be obtained in UK from Swiss Serum and Vaccine Institute through a pharmaceutical importer.

Rabies (p. 232)
Freeze-dried inactivated vaccine cultured on human diploid cells. Pre-exposure vaccination recommended for travellers to remote rabies enzootic areas where post-exposure treatment unlikely to be available and for persons exposed to risk of infection.

Tick-borne encephalitis (p. 70)
Inactivated vaccine prepared from virus grown in chick embryo. Recommended for travellers likely to be exposed to tick bites in forest areas of Central Europe, especially Austria and Russia.

Typhoid (p. 251)
- Vaccine: heat-killed, phenol-preserved, *Salm. typhi* whole-cell vaccine. Paratyphoid vaccines of unproven value.
- Dose: primary immunization two doses 0.5 ml deep subcutaneous or i.m. injection, 4–6 weeks apart (0.25 ml for children 1–10 years); reinforcing dose every 3 years under continued exposure. Intradermal injection is not recommended for primary immunization but may be used for reinforcing doses.
- Recommendations: residents of, and travellers to, endemic areas where conditions of hygiene and sanitation are poor, includes areas in most countries outside Australasia, Europe and North America; laboratory workers handling cultures or specimens which may contain *Salm. typhi*.

• Contraindications: not recommended for children under 1 year of age because of low incidence at this age.

Yellow fever (pp. 327, 333)
• Vaccine: live-attenuated, freeze-dried vaccine (17D-strain virus). Available from vaccination centres; in UK see DHSS leaflet SA40 *Travellers' Guide to Health* (published annually).
• Dose: single injection 0.5 ml deep subcutaneous.
• Recommendations: international certificate valid from 10 days after injection for 10 years; valid immediately after revaccination; usually compulsory for endemic areas of Central Africa and South America; compulsory for entry to some Asian countries in travellers from or through endemic areas.
• Contraindications: infants under 9 months because of very rare encephalitis, unless exposure to infection unavoidable; pregnant women because of theoretical risk of fetal infection, unless risk of yellow fever outweighs this theoretical risk.

Other vaccines

Anthrax (p. 8)
• Vaccine: alum-precipitated antigen from sterile cell-free filtrate of Sterne-strain cultures of *Bacillus anthracis*.
• Dose: primary course — three doses 0.5 ml i.m. at intervals of 3 weeks with fourth dose after 6 months; annual reinforcing dose whilst exposure continues.
• Recommendation: workers exposed to risk of anthrax.
• Contraindications: see general contraindications (p. 355).

Hepatitis B (p. 120)
• Vaccines: purified, formalin-inactivated, alum-adsorbed hepatitis B surface antigen (HBsAg) prepared from human plasma; HBsAg prepared in yeast cells by recombinant DNA technique.
• Dose: primary course of three doses containing 20 µg HBsAg, i.m. injection into deltoid, the second and third doses at intervals of 1 month and 6 months; need for reinforcing doses not yet established; may be given intradermally in persons over 10 years but immune

response should be confirmed by a post immunization serological test.

● Recommendations: health-care personnel and laboratory staff who have direct contact with blood or body fluids of patients; patients admitted to mental handicap units where there is a high prevalence of hepatitis B infection; family contacts of carriers; infants born to carrier mothers (p. 127); haemophiliacs and recipients of multiple blood transfusions; other persons who will be exposed to the blood or body fluids of carriers.

● Contraindications: see general contraindications (p. 355)

Influenza (p. 143)

● Vaccine: whole-cell, split-virus or surface-antigen vaccine prepared from virus grown in chick embryo; formulation changed annually to include recently circulating strains of virus. Recommendations published by WHO.

● Dose: single dose, deep subcutaneous or i.m. injection, annually for persons at special risk.

● Recommendations: persons with chronic heart, lung or renal disease, diabetes and patients in whom immunosupressive therapy is proposed; should be considered for residents in old people's homes. Not recommended under 4 years of age. Repeat annual immunization of healthy persons in closed communities, such as schools, has been advocated but it is not established that this gives a high level of protection. Immunization of health-care staff should be considered if epidemic is anticipated.

● Contraindications: see general contraindications (p. 355); whole-cell vaccines should not be given to children under 15 years.

Pneumococcal infection (pp. 212, 289)

● Vaccine: polyvalent capsular polysaccharide vaccine prepared from 23 types of pneumococci.

● Dose: single injection, deep subcutaneous or i.m.

● Recommendations: persons at high risk of developing pneumococcal disease, e.g. patients with splenic dysfunction, prior to splenectomy, patients with chronic cardiorespiratory disease. Not recommended under 2 years of age because of poor antibody response.

● Contraindications: should not be given to patients who have had previous injection of pneumococcal vaccine.

Passive immunization
Passive immunity may be acquired naturally by fetus from mother or by infant from colostrum or milk; usually protects for about 6 months. Artificial passive immunity can be induced by i.m. injection of pre-formed antibody from humans or animals; has immediate effect but limited duration.

Administration
● Adrenaline injection 1 : 1000 and hydrocortisone must be available.
● Give test dose for systemic reaction before injection of non-human antitoxin.
● Intramuscular or deep subcutaneous injection after ensuring needle point is not in small blood vessel.
● Large doses of human immunoglobulin should be divided and given in several sites.
● Observe patient for half an hour after non-human antitoxin so that anaphylaxis may be treated promptly.

Human normal immunoglobulin
Derived from pooled donor blood. Recommended for measles, post-exposure prophylaxis in debilitated children and immunocompromised (p. 172), for pre-exposure hepatitis A prophylaxis for travellers to insanitary areas, post-exposure prophylaxis for household and institutional contacts (pp. 126–7), and for rubella post-exposure prophylaxis in non-immune pregnant women, but only indicated if termination unlikely to be accepted (p. 244).

Human specific immunoglobulin
Derived from blood of selected donors with high antibody titres.
● *Chickenpox*: zoster immunoglobulin (ZIG), prophylaxis in neonates and immunocompromised (p. 324).
● *Hepatitis B*: hepatitis B immunoglobulin (HBIG), post-exposure prophylaxis following accidental inoculation of blood from case or carrier; infants of mothers with hepatitis B (p. 127).

Appendix C: Immunization

- *Rabies*: human rabies immunoglobulin (HRIG), part of post-exposure treatment (p. 234).
- *Tetanus*: human tetanus immunoglobin (HTIG), prophylaxis in wound management and treatment of tetanus (p. 293).

Antitoxins prepared in animals
- *Botulism*: equine antitoxin, prophylaxis in persons suspected of eating contaminated food (p. 93), and treatment (p. 84)
- *Diphtheria*: equine antitoxin, in treatment (p. 59)

Index

abattoir workers *see* butchers, abattoir workers and meat handlers
abortion and: anaerobic infections, 5; chlamydial infection, 32; HIV infection, 44; listeriosis, 157; parvovirus infection, 206; rubella, 244; sepsis, 222−224; syphilis, 300; toxoplasmosis, 297
acanthamoeba, infection of eye, 49
acrodermatitis chronica atrophicans, 161
actinomycosis, 1−2
acquired immune deficiency syndrome (Aids), 136
adenovirus and: conjunctivitis, 47−49; enteritis, 99; respiratory infection, 238
agricultural workers *see* farmers
Aids-related complex (ARC), 135
amylase in mumps, 187
anaerobic infections, 3−7
anthrax, 8−9
antitoxins in: botulism, 84, 93; diphtheria, 59; tetanus, 292−293 *see also* passive immunization, 364−365
appendicitis and: actinomycosis, 1−2; campylobacter, 95; measles, 172; yersinia, 340
Argentine haemorrhagic fever, 329−330
arthritis and arthralgia, 11−14 *see also* bacillary dysentery, 64; brucellosis, 19; campylobacter, 95; chlamydiae, 30; erysipeloid, 259; *H. influenzae*, 113; hepatitis B, 123−124; HIV infection, 134; Kawasaki disease, 148; Lyme disease, 161; meningococcal disease 11−12, 183; mumps, 187; mycobacteria, 14; *N. gonorrhoeae*, 13−14; paratyphoid, 253; parvovirus infection, 12, 205; rheumatic fever, 282; rubella, 242; salmonella infections, 12; syphilis, 301; yersinia infections, 12, 340
aspergillosis, 15−17: and endocarditis, 75

athlete's foot, 262
atypical mycobacterial infections, 196−198
atypical pneumonia, 215−217

Bacillus cereus and: food poisoning, 86−87; wound infection, 86
bacteraemia and: actinomycosis, 1; anaerobes, non-sporing, 4, 223; anthrax, 9; brucellosis, 19; clostridia, 6, 223; endocarditis, 73−75; enterococci, 233; erysipelas, 281; erysipeloid, 259; gonococci, 107; listeriosis, 157−158; meningitis, 180; meningococci, 183; plague, 337; salmonellae, 248, 251, 253; sepsis, post-abortum and post-partum, 222−223; *Sh. dysenteriae*, 64; *Staph. aureus*, 223, 274; streptococci group B, 286; *Str. pneumoniae*, 213; *Str. pyogenes*, 222, 278, 281; tularaemia, 307; urinary tract infection, 316; *Y. enterocolitica*, 340
BCG and: leprosy, 201; tuberculosis, 195, 358
bilharziasis *see* schistosomiasis, 66
Black Death, 337
blackwater fever, 165
blood transfusion and: cytomegalovirus, 54; hepatitis B, 128; HIV, 133; malaria, 168
Bolivian haemorrhagic fever, 329−330
boomerang leg, 305
Bornholm disease, 79−80
botulism, 83−84: wound, 5
boutonneuse fever, 309
brain abscess and: actinomycosis, 2; anaerobes, non-sporing, 4; aspergillosis, 16; *E. histolytica*, 62; *Staph. aureus*, 274
Brazilian purpuric fever, 48
Brill−Zinsser disease, 311
brucellosis, 18−20
butchers, abattoir workers and meat handlers, infection in: anthrax, 8; brucellosis, 18; cowpox, 265;

erysipeloid, 259; impetigo, 257; orf and paravaccinia, 265; Q fever, 229; streptococcal infection, 288

campylobacter enteritis, 94−96
cancrum oris, 238
candida infections, 21−23
canicola fever, 154−155
carcinoma and HIV infection, 137
carcinoma of cervix and: herpes simplex, 129, genital warts, 265
cat-scratch fever, 24−25
cerebral abscess see brain abscess
chancre, 300
chancroid, 26−27: and HIV, 26
Charcot−Leyden crystals, 62
chemoprophylaxis, 342−345
see also anaerobic infections, 7; anthrax, 9; chlamydial infection, 32; cholera, 37; diphtheria, 60; endocarditis, 343; herpes simplex, 44, 132; influenza, 145; Lassa fever, 335; leprosy, 201; listeriosis, 45, 159; malaria, 168; meningitis, 114, 185, 344; plague, 339; post-splenectomy patients, 344; rheumatic fever, 282; scrub typhus, 313; streptococci group B infections, 43−44, 287; tetanus, 292; urinary infections, 319
chickenpox (varicella), 321−324
Chikungunya fever, 326
chlamydial infections, 28−34
cholera, 35−37
colitis: haemorrhagic, 38−39; necrotizing in infants, 39−40; pseudomembranous, 40−42; and *Staph. aureus*, 274; and *Y. enterocolitica*, 340
common cold, 238
congenital and neonatal infections, 43−46
see also bacteria, Gram-negative, 43; chlamydiae, 30; conjunctivitis, 49; cytomegalovirus, 52−53; hepatitis B, 122; herpes simplex, 131; HIV, 134; listeriosis, 157; malaria, 163; necrotizing enterocolitis, 39−40; rubella, 241;
streptococci group B, 285; syphilis, 301; toxoplasmosis, 295; varicella, 321, 324
conjunctivitis, 47−51
see also adenovirus, 238; chlamydial, 28, 30; diphtheritic, 58; enterovirus, 78; gonococcal, 107; herpes simplex, 130; inclusion, 30; Kawasaki disease, 147; listeria, 158; measles, 171; pharyngo-conjunctival fever, 238; phlyctenular, 191; *Staph. aureus*, 274; *Str. pneumoniae*, 289
containment isolation, 348−351
coronary artery disease, in Kawasaki disease, 148
corticosteroids in: colitis, pseudomembranous, 42; hepatitis, 126; infectious mononucleosis, 142; leprosy, 201; measles, 172; PUO, 228; rheumatic fever, 282; trichiniasis, 119; toxoplasmosis, 297; typhoid fever, 254
cowpox, 265−266
Creutzfeldt−Jakob disease, 70, 71
Crimean−Congo haemorrhagic fever, 327
croup, 239
Cryptococcus neoformans: encephalitis, 137; meningitis, 174, 177
cutaneous infections see skin infections
cutaneous larva migrans, 118
cytomegalovirus infection, 52−54

dairy products, transmission in: brucellosis, 18; haemorrhagic colitis, 38; diphtheria, 57; campylobacter enteritis, 95; *E. coli*, 97; cryptosporidiosis, 102; dysentery, 64; listeriosis, 157; Q fever, 229; salmonellosis, 247; typhoid and paratyphoid, 251; staphylococcal food poisoning, 85; streptococcal infections, 278; tuberculosis, 190; yersinia infection, 339

deafness and: meningitis, 183;
rubella, 243; typhus, 310
dengue, 55–56, 326
dengue-like fever, 326
dermatitis, seborrhoeic and HIV
infection, 135
see also skin infections
dermatophytes, 262
diphtheria, 57–60
disseminated intravascular
coagulation (DIC) and: dengue, 56;
Lassa fever, 329; meningococcal
infection, 183; plague, 337; typhus,
310
drug abusers, infection in: anaerobic
infections, 3, 5; botulism, 5;
hepatitis B, 121; HIV infection, 133;
endocarditis, 74; malaria, 163;
pseudomonas infection, 13;
tetanus, 290
dysentery: amoebic, 61–63; bacillary,
64–66; schistosomal, 66–68

Ebola virus infection, 331
eczema: herpeticum, 130;
vaccinatum, 265, 267
encephalitis, 69–72
see also: amoebic, primary, 71;
candidiasis, 22; cat-scratch fever,
24; cryptococcal, 137;
cytomegalovirus infection, 137;
herpes simplex, 131; HIV infection,
134; infectious mononucleosis,
141; influenza, 145; Lyme disease,
161; measles, 170–172; mumps,
187; Rift Valley fever, 327, 333;
rubella, 242; SSPE, 170, 172;
toxoplasmosis, 137, 296; varicella
and herpes zoster, 322, 323; Weil's
disease, 154
endocarditis, 73–76
see also: anaerobes, non-sporing,
4; aspergillosis, 16; candida, 22;
erysipeloid, 259; gonococcal, 107;
Q fever, 230; rheumatic 282;
salmonella, 248; streptococci,
286, 288
enteric fever, 250–256
enterovirus infections, 77–82

eosinophilia and: dysentery,
schistosomal, 68; helminths,
common intestinal, 116–119; PUO,
227
epidermal necrolysis, 273
epiglottitis, 113, 239
erysipelas, 258, 280–281
erysipeloid, 259–260
erythema chronicum migrans, 161
erythema infectiosum (fifth disease),
205
erythema nodosum in: leprosy, 200;
tuberculosis, 191; *Y. enterocolitica*
infection, 340
Escherichia coli in: gastroenteritis,
96–98; haemolytic uraemic
syndrome, 110; haemorrhagic
colitis, 38; pneumonia, 212; urinary
tract infection, 315
exotoxins in: *B. anthracis*, 8;
Clostridium spp., 5, 40, 41, 83, 290;
C. diphtheriae, 57; *Sh. dysenteriae*,
64; *Staph. aureus*, 271; *Str.
pyogenes*, 277; *V. cholerae*, 35

farmers, infection in: actinomycosis,
1; anthrax, 8; brucellosis, 18;
chlamydial, 32; cowpox, 265;
erysipeloid, 259; leptospirosis, 153;
listeriosis, 157; Newcastle virus
conjunctivitis, 49; orf and
paravaccinia, 265; Q fever, 229;
streptococcal, 288
fifth disease, 205
fish and infection: botulism, 83;
erysipeloid, 259; leptospirosis, 153;
V. parahaemolyticus, 89
fish, toxic poisoning, 91
fleas and: plague, 336; typhus, 309
foodborne infection: anthrax, 8;
botulism, 83; campylobacter, 95;
cholera, 35; colitis, haemorrhagic,
38; cryptosporidiosis, 102;
dysentery, 61, 64; *E. coli*, 97; food
poisoning, 83–93; gastroenteritis,
viral, 90, 99; haemolytic uraemic
syndrome, 110; hepatitis A, 122;
Lassa fever, 330; leptospirosis, 153;

listeriosis, 157; roundworm, 115; salmonellosis, 246; small round viruses, 90; streptococci, 278; toxoplasmosis, 295; trichiniasis, 119; tularaemia, 307; typhoid and paratyphoid, 251; whipworm, 116; yersinia, 339
   see also dairy products

food handlers as source of infection: hepatitis A, 122; salmonellosis, 247; staphylococcal food poisoning, 85; typhoid and paratyphoid, 251; viral gastroenteritis, 99

food poisoning: bacterial, 83–90; chemical, 91–92; prevention, 92–93; viral, 90–91

furuncle, 273

gangosa, 305

gas gangrene, 5–6

gastroenteritis, 94–103: and salmonellosis, 247

genital infection: anaerobic, 3, 4, 222; candida, 21; chancroid, 26; gonococcal, 106; herpes simplex, 129; HIV, 133; listeriosis, 157; non-specific, 28, 207; pelvic inflammatory disease, 207; streptococcal, 222, 286; syphilis, 299; toxic shock syndrome, 274

German measles, 241–245

Ghon focus, 190

giardiasis, 104–105

glandular fever *see* infectious mononucleosis, 140–142

glomerulonephritis, 282–283

gonorrhoea, 106–109: associated with chlamydiae, 29

gumma, 301

haemolytic uraemic syndrome, 110–111

Haemophilus influenzae infections, 112–114
   see also arthritis, 13, 113; meningitis, 179; osteomyelitis, 202

haemorrhagic fevers, viral, 325–335

hand, foot and mouth disease, 80

Heaf test, 195

health-care staff and infection: anaerobic, 3; diphtheria, 356; dysentery, 66; hepatitis B, 121, 363; herpes simplex, 129; HIV, 134, 139; influenza, 146, 363; Lassa fever, 330; Marburg/Ebola virus diseases, 332; meningococcal infection, 185; paratyphoid fever, 255; pertussis, 211; poliomyelitis, 81, 357; rabies, 235; rubella, 245; salmonellosis, 249; tuberculosis, 359; typhoid fever, 255; varicella, 324

helminth infections, 115–119

hepatitis: cytomegalovirus, 53; delta agent, 120; Epstein–Barr virus, 140; non-A non-B, 121; Q fever, 230; syphilis, 301; toxoplasmosis, 296; virus A, 120; virus B, 120; Weil's disease, 154; yellow fever, 325

herpangina, 80

herpes simplex infections, 129–132

herpes zoster (shingles), 321–324

hide porters' disease, 8

HIV, 133–139

HLA-B27 and arthritis, 11, 340

hookworm infection, 117

human immunodeficiency virus (HIV) infection, 133–139

immunization, active, 352–364: administration of vaccines, 352; childhood immunization, 355; contraindications, 353; for travel, 359; side effects, 354; storage of vaccines, 352
   see also anthrax, 362; cholera, 360; diphtheria, 60, 356; encephalitis, tick-borne, 361; hepatitis B, 362; HIV-infected persons, 139; influenza, 146, 363; Japanese B encephalitis, 360; leprosy, 201; measles, 357; meningococcal infection, 360; mumps, 358; pertussis, 211, 355; plague, 360; pneumococcal, 363; poliomyelitis, 357; rabies, 234, 361; rubella, 244,

358; tetanus, 293, 357; tuberculosis, 195, 358; typhoid fever, 255, 256, 361; typhus, louse-borne, 361; yellow fever, 362
immunization, passive, 364–365
see also botulism, 93; hepatitis A, 126–127; hepatitis B, 127; measles, 172; rabies, 234; rubella, 244; tetanus, 293; varicella, 324
immunodeficiency and: anaerobic infections, 4; arthritis, suppurative, 12; aspergillosis, 15; candidiasis, 22; cryptococcosis, 137, 176; cryptosporidium, 101, 102; cytomegalovirus, 53; herpes simplex, 129, 131; herpes zoster, 321; HIV infection, 133–139; immunization, 353; listeriosis, 157; measles, 170, 172; mycobacteria, 136; pneumonia, 212; *P. carinii*, 219; *Staph. epidermidis*, 272; toxoplasmosis, 295; varicella, 321
immunoglobulins *see* immunization, passive, 364–365
impetigo, 257, 273, 281
inclusion conjunctivitis, 30
infection control, 346–351
infectious mononucleosis, 140–142
influenza A and B, 143–146
intravascular haemolysis and clostridia, 6
isolation: containment, 349; high-security, 350; strict, 350
isospora infection, 136
IUCD and: actinomycosis, 1; chemoprophylaxis, 343; pelvic inflammatory disease, 207

Jakob–Creutzfeldt encephalitis, 70, 71
Japanese B encephalitis, 70, 360

Kaposi's sarcoma, 137
Katayama fever, 67
Kawasaki disease, 147–148
keratitis and: acanthamoeba, 49; aspergillosis, 16; herpes zoster, 323
kerion, 263
Koplik's spots, 171

Korean haemorrhagic fever, 328
kuru, 70, 71
Kyasanur Forest disease, 328

laboratory workers, infection in: arbovirus encephalitis, 70; chlamydial infection, 32; cytomegalovirus, 54; hepatitis B, 121, 362; Lassa fever, 330; lymphocytic choriomeningitis, 174; Marburg/Ebola virus, 332; nephropathia epidemica, 328; Q fever, 229; rabies, 235; tuberculosis, 358; tularaemia, 307; typhoid fever, 255, 361; *Y. pestis*, 336, 361
lactose intolerance, 98
Lassa fever, 329–330
legionnaires disease, 149, 152
lepromin test, 200
leprosy, 198–201
leptospirosis, 153–156
leucoplakia, hairy, 135
lice, head and body, 268: and typhus, 309
listeriosis, 157–159
see also congenital and neonatal infection, 45; meningitis, 179
liver abscess: amoebic, 62; and anaerobes, non-sporing, 4
Loeffler's syndrome, 116
Lyme disease, 160–162
lymphadenitis benigna cutis, 161
lymphogranuloma venereum (LGV), 28–29
lymphoma: and HIV infection, 137; non-Hodgkin's, 137

malaria, 163–169: and prophylaxis 168
Mantoux test, 195
Marburg disease, 331
measles, 170–173
meningitis, 174–181
see also amoebic, 71; anaerobes, non-sporing, 4; bacteria, Gram-negative, 41; candida, 22; canicola fever, 155; cryptococcal, 177; enterovirus, 78; gonococcal,

107; *H. influenzae*, 113; herpes
simplex, 131; herpes zoster, 323;
HIV, 135; infectious mononucleosis, 141; influenza, 145;
Kawasaki disease, 148;
leptospirosis, 154, 155, 176; listeria,
158; Lyme disease, 161;
lymphocytic choriomeningitis, 174;
meningococcal, 183; mumps, 187;
neonatal, 180; plague, 337;
poliovirus, 78; salmonella, 248;
streptococci group B, 285; *Strep.
pneumoniae*, 213; syphilis, 301;
tuberculous, 191; tularaemia, 307;
Weil's disease, 154
meningococcal infection, 182–185
metallic poisoning, 92
milkborne infection *see* dairy
products
mites and: scabies, 368; typhus, 309
molluscum contagiosum, 265, 266
mosquitoes and: chikungunya fever,
326; dengue, 55, 326; equine
encephalitis, 70; Japanese B
encephalitis, 70; malaria, 163; Rift
Valley fever, 327; yellow fever, 327
mucocutaneous lymph node
syndrome *see* Kawasaki disease,
147–148
mumps, 186–188
mushroom poisoning, 92
mycobacterial infections, 189–201
see also arthritis, 13; HIV infection,
136; meningitis, 175, 177;
osteomyelitis, 202
mycoplasma infections, 216–217
myocarditis and: diphtheria, 58;
Kawasaki disease, 147; Lyme
disease, 161; mumps, 187; *M.
pneumoniae*, 217; trichiniasis, 119;
typhoid fever, 253

nappy rash, candida, 22
necrolysis, acute epidermal, 273
necrotizing enterocolitis, 39
Negri bodies, 232, 233
neonatal infection *see* congenital and
neonatal infections

nephritis and: cytomegalovirus
infection, 52; endocarditis, 73;
infectious mononucleosis, 141;
leptospirosis, 154; malaria, 165;
streptococcal infections, 282–283
nephropathia epidemica (Korean
haemorrhagic fever), 328
neuropathy, diphtheritic, 58
Nikolsky's sign, 273
notifiable infectious diseases in
England and Wales, 346

Omsk haemorrhagic fever, 328
ophthalmia neonatorum: chlamydial,
28, 30; gonococcal, 49, 107
orchitis and: Bornholm disease, 80;
mumps, 187
orf, 265
ornithosis, 32–34
osteomyelitis, 202–204
otitis externa and: aspergillosis, 16;
pseudomonas infection, 261
otitis media, 238; and: anaerobes,
non-sporing, 4; *H. influenzae*, 113;
Kawasaki disease, 148; measles,
172; *Str. pneumoniae*, 289; *Str.
pyogenes*, 280, 281

pancreatitis in mumps, 187
paratyphoid fever, 250–256
paravaccinia, 265, 266
paronychia and: candida, 22; *Staph.
aureus*, 273
parotitis in mumps, 187
parvovirus B19 infections, 205–206
see also arthritis, 12; congenital
infection, 45
Paul–Bunnell test, 53
pediculosis, 268–270
pelvic inflammatory disease,
207–208: and actinomycosis, 1;
chlamydial, 28; gonococcal, 107
pertussis, 209–211
pets and infection: campylobacter,
95; cat-scratch fever, 24;
cryptosporidiosis, 102;
leptospirosis, 153; mycobacterial
ulcer, 196; plague, 336; psittacosis,
32; rabies, 232; rickettsial

infection, 309; ringworm, 262;
salmonellosis, 246; toxoplasmosis,
295; vaccinia, 265; yersiniosis, 339
pharyngoconjunctival fever, 48, 238
'pigbel', 88
plague, 336–338
pneumonia, 212–231
see also: anthrax, 9; aspergillosis,
15; candida, 22; Chl. trachomatis,
30; cytomegalovirus, 53;
H. influenzae, 113; HIV infection,
136; influenza, 145; klebsiella, 214;
legionnaires disease, 150;
lymphoid interstitial, 136;
mycoplasmal, 216; ornithosis, 33;
pertussis, 210; plague, 337;
pneumococcal, 289; P. carinii, 136;
Q fever, 229–230; staphylococcal
274; Str. pyogenes, 281;
toxoplasmosis, 296; varicella, 322
poliomyelitis, 77–82
Pontiac fever, 152
post-abortum and post-partum
sepsis, 222–224
post-viral fatigue syndrome and:
Coxsackie virus, 77; infectious
mononucleosis, 141
psittacosis, 32–34
puerperal fever, 222
pyrexia of undetermined origin
(PUO), 225–228

Q fever, 229–231

rabies, 232–236: immunization, 235,
361; post-exposure treatment,
234–235
red kidney bean poisoning, 92
Reiter's disease, 29, 317
respiratory infections (acute),
237–240
Reye's syndrome, 143, 145
rheumatic fever, 281–282
Rift Valley fever, 327
ringworm, 262
Rocky Mountain spotted fever, 309,
311–312
rose spots and: ornithosis, 33;
typhoid and paratyphoid, 252

roundworm infection, 115–116
rubella, 241–245: immunization, 244,
358

salmonellosis, 246–250
scabies, 269
scalded-skin syndrome, 273
scarlet fever, 278–280
Schick test, 356
schistosomiasis, 66–68
scrumpox, 257
septicaemia see bacteraemia
shellfish and infection: cholera, 35;
hepatitis A, 122; typhoid fever, 251;
toxic, 92; V. parahaemolyticus, 89;
viral gastroenteritis, 99
shigella infections see dysentery
shingles see herpes zoster, 321–324
shipyard workers' eye, 48
sickle-cell disease and: malaria, 164;
parvovirus infection, 206;
salmonella osteomyelitis, 202
sinusitis, 238
see also anaerobes, non-sporing, 4;
aspergillosis, 16; H. influenzae, 113;
Str. pyogenes, 280
skin infections, 257–268
see also actinomycosis, 1; anthrax,
8; candida, 22; diphtheria, 58;
hand, foot and mouth disease, 78,
80; herpes simplex, 130; leprosy,
198; mycobacterial ulcers, 197;
staphylococcal, 273; streptococcal,
280, 288; synergistic bacterial
gangrene, 288; syphilis, 300; yaws,
304
skin infestations, 268–270
slapped-cheek syndrome, 205
slim disease, 137
slow virus infections, 69
staphylococcal infections, 271–276
see also arthritis, 12; conjunctivitis,
49; endocarditis, 74; food
poisoning, 85–86; impetigo, 257;
meningitis, 179; osteomyelitis, 202;
pneumonia, 214, 274; post-abortum
and post-partum sepsis, 222
stomatitis, 238: candida, 21; herpes
simplex, 130

streptococcus, group B infections, 285–287
  see also congenital and neonatal infections, 43; post-abortum and post-partum sepsis, 222
streptococcus (other) infections, 287–289
  see also meningitis, 179; otitis media, 238; pneumonia, 214
Streptococcus pyogenes infections, 277–284
  see also impetigo, 257–258; osteomyelitis, 202–204; post-abortum and post-partum sepsis, 222–224
swimming, infections associated with: conjunctivitis, 28, 47; legionnaires disease, 149; leptospirosis, 153; meningo-encephalitis, primary amoebic, 71; pharyngoconjunctival fever, 48; plantar warts, 266; swimmer's ear, 261; swimmer's itch, 67; 'swimming pool granuloma', 196; 'swimming pool rash', 260; tinea pedis, 262
sycosis barbae, 273
syphilis, 299–303

tenosynovitis: gonococcal, 13; rubella, 12; tuberculous, 14
tetanus, 290–294
threadworm infection, 115
thrush, 21
ticks and: Crimean–Congo haemorrhagic fever, 327; encephalitis, 70, 361; Kyasanur Forest disease, 328; Lyme disease, 160; Omsk haemorrhagic fever, 328; Q fever, 229; tularaemia, 307; typhus, 309
tinea infections, 262–265
T-lymphocytes and HIV infection, 134
tonsillitis, 238
  see also diphtheritic, 58; enteroviruses, 79–80; gonococcal, 107; infectious mononucleosis, 141; streptococcal, 279

toxic food poisoning: botulism, 83; chemical, 91; staphylococcal, 85
toxic shock syndrome, 274
toxoplasmosis, 295–298
trachoma, 28–30
traveller's diarrhoea: campylobacter enteritis, 94; dysentery, 64; *E. coli* enteritis, 97; giardiasis, 104; salmonellosis, 246
treponemal infections, 299–306
trichiniasis, 119
tropical splenomegaly syndrome and malaria, 165
tuberculosis, 189–196
  see also arthritis, 13, 14; meningitis, 175, 177; osteomyelitis, 202–204
tularaemia, 307–308
typhoid and paratyphoid fevers, 250–256
typhus, 309–314

urethritis, 217: chlamydial (non-gonococcal), 29; gonococcal, 107; in Kawasaki disease, 148; in listeriosis, 158
urinary tract infections, 315–320; and: candida, 22; *Staph. epidermidis*, 273; streptococcus group B, 286

vaccinia, 267
vagabond's disease, 269
varicella (chickenpox), 321–324
verotoxin, 96, 110
veterinarians, infection in: anthrax, 8, 9; brucellosis, 18–19; listeriosis, 157; Q fever, 229; rabies, 235
viral haemorrhagic fevers, 325–335

waterborne infections: campylobacter, 95; cholera, 35; cryptosporidiosis, 102; dysentery, 61, 64; giardiasis, 104; hepatitis, A/non-A non-B, 122; leptospirosis, 153; toxoplasmosis, 295; tularaemia, 307; typhoid fever, 251
warts, 265–268
wasting syndrome, 137

Waterhouse–Friderichsen syndrome,
183
Weil's disease, 153–156
whipworm infection, 116
whitlow, herpetic, 130
whooping cough (pertussis), 209–211

yaws, 304–306
yellow fever, 327
yersinia infections, 336–341
    see also arthritis, 11, 12; plague,
    336–339

zoonoses, arthropod-borne:
    boutonneuse fever, 309; Lyme
    disease, 160; plague, 326; typhus,
    309; viral haemorrhagic fevers, 325

zoonoses, food, milk or waterborne:
    brucellosis, 18; campylobacter
    infection, 94; cryptosporidiosis,
    101; diphtheria, 57; giardiasis, 104;
    haemolytic uraemic syndrome, 110;
    haemorrhagic colitis, 98; listeriosis,
    157; salmonellosis, 246; *Strep.
    zooepidemicus*, 287; trichiniasis,
    119; tuberculosis, 189; tularaemia,
    307; yersiniosis, 336
zoonoses, occupationally-acquired:
    see butchers, abattoir workers and
    meat handlers; farmers; laboratory
    workers; veterinarians
zoonoses, pet-associated see pets
zoster immunoglobulin (ZIG), 43, 324,
364